THANK YOU FOR JOINING ME,
I'm so excited for you!

Hi, I'm Michelle, author of The Empowered Eating Handbook and creator of the Empowered Eating Course and Workbook.

My journey began when I was very young and fought my own health battles. In addition, having spent my childhood so-called "overweight" and "different" I was the target of abuse from my peers and was unable to see my true worth until much later in my journey.

Sometimes, I feel like I've been on a diet my entire life. I certainly know what it's like to battle with the ups and downs of poor health, diet confusion, and low self-esteem. I know what it's like to be a slave to the scale and ride the yo-yo diet roller coaster.

But I've broken free, regained my health (and sanity) and this workbook and my course will help you to do the same.

I did receive some formal training too!

I received my bachelor degree at Dalhousie University, Halifax while later achieving a graduate degree in education at the University of Maine at Fort Kent. I then furthered my nutrition education with a Graduate Certificate in Holistic Performance Nutrition from The Holistic Performance Institute and a registered Health Coach through HCANZA.

Recently I completed my training to become a "The Body Positive" facilitator and am also a licensed Am I Hungry?™ Mindful Eating instructor. I have also studied the 'non-diet approach' and intuitive eating with Evelyn Tribole co-author of *Intuitive Eating*.

I can't wait to work with you.

Learn more at www.michelleyandle.com

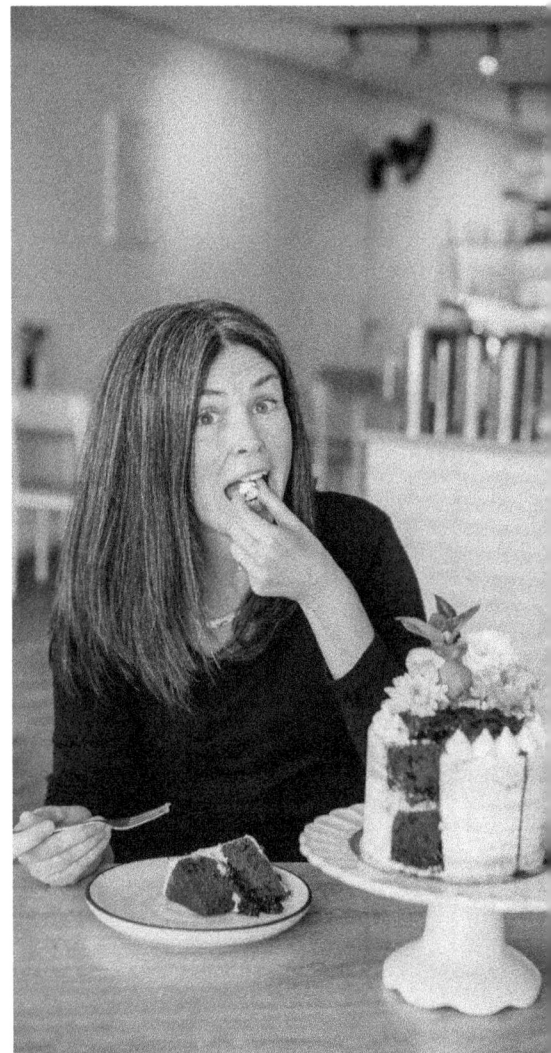

Michelle Yandle

THE EMPOWERED EATING

WORKBOOK

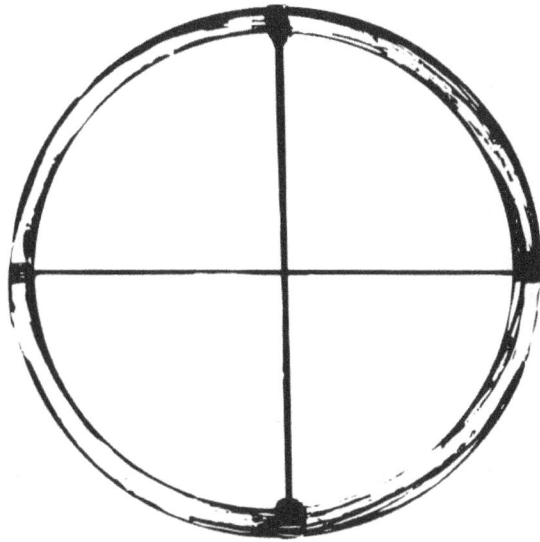

Learning to be your healthest self without giving up the foods you love.

INTRODUCTION

I'll never forget the 60-year-old woman who walked into my office too scared to eat a bowl of porridge. This is despite the fact that there was once a time when she'd eaten a bowl of porridge every morning. It fuelled her and satisfied her. She would be content for hours without needing anything else to eat. But she read somewhere that she shouldn't eat oats, that they were too high in carbs and would make her fat.

I asked her, whether she was "overweight"* when she used to eat oats?

To which she replied that she hadn't been - and logic struck.

And so, there lies the problem. We've made something so inherently natural, the act of feeding and nourishing ourselves, utterly confusing. We've lost our natural ability to simply listen to our body's messages. Meanwhile, we're so afraid of 'fat' that we're willing to compromise our health in order to avoid it or lose it.

We all know that person, the one who can 'eat whatever they want' without worry. If they are not hungry, they may turn down the chocolate cake. If they are not hungry, they might even skip a meal. If they want the cheesecake, they have it and enjoy it. But gasp! They may not even finish it!

There was a time in history when we are all eating "instinctively" and in a way that simply made us feel good. In my opinion, eating to feel good and being able to listen to our bodies are the missing pieces of the puzzle, when our physical, mental and spiritual health is at stake. Empowered Eating will help you to do both.

*The term 'overweight" is not actually helpful. Over what weight? We'll dig more into this in the second principle.

MY STORY

Sometimes, I feel like I've been on a diet my entire life.

I don't quite remember when it all started, but I did grow up in a home where I watched the beautiful women in my life consistently strive to lose weight. I watched my sister and my mother, two of the most intelligent and amazing people I know, struggle with their own dieting roller coaster ride. I think it would have started for me around the age of 9 or 10 as I can vividly remember asking my mother around that time whether or not I would get fat if I ate too many oranges.

I then hopped on the diet roller coaster myself and didn't manage to get off for a very long time. By the time I was 14 I had been on as many diets as I was old. Weight Watchers, Nutrisystem, SlimFast, Richard Simmons (my personal favourite) and all of them in between.

I grew up hating my body, and the teasing at school didn't help. Being 'different', not fitting the socially accepted mould, meant years of bullying, teasing and taunting further propelling me into the downward spiral of the dieting industry.

When I was about 15, something 'miraculous' happened. I lost weight, and it was staying off. I was skinny! Hoorah!! But I realise now, so many years later that the weight may have come off physically but I held onto it mentally for most of my life.

I would still look in the mirror and see flaws. I would still look at my tiny arms and think they were fat. I would poke and prod and count my flaws every time I got the chance. I felt unloveable, imperfect, and for many years, turned to alcohol as a way to have a bit of confidence.

The weight never really did come back on, but the feelings I had for myself continued to throw me into every 'healthy diet' you could imagine. I used these plans and programs as ways of getting 'healthy' when ultimately it was simply a tool to make sure the weight never came back because the very thought terrified me.

I tried it all, raw diets, paleo diets, macrobiotic, juice fasts, sugar-free, carb-free, you name it. I've done it. I don't think there is a type of food out there that I haven't quit at one point or another. I pretended these diets were just healthy eating. But then things became obsessive, I began to fear certain foods, and over time, my health suffered. I didn't even realise it at the time. After all, I was just eating healthily.

My "ah-ha" moment didn't come until a few years later. While I was studying nutrition, I wrote an article for my school on orthorexia. It was called, "When healthy eating goes too far". I wanted to educate people on what can happen when we become obsessive. I read the story to my husband, feeling very proud of my achievement. Upon finishing it he said to me "So, you're writing about yourself?" Though I didn't realise it at the time, those words changed my life for the better. Writing that paper was the best thing that ever happened to my health.

I've since started with a clean slate. I now read things with a critical eye and sort facts from fiction. I've tuned into the simplistic wisdom of my ancestors and learned to listen to the messages inside me. I feel like I've regained a long lost friend and have never felt better physically and mentally. It's a liberating experience to be able to eat the foods I love while still nurturing my body. I'm the one in charge now, I'm the expert on what my body needs each day, and I feel fantastic.

So how did a chronic yo-yo dieter finally learn to eat instinctively? By using many of the tools in this workbook. I'm not perfect, I'm a work in progress, but as long as I continue to take the steps needed to be in charge of my thoughts and actions, I'm heading in the right direction and so can you.

I want to gift this to you all. I want you all to feel liberated too, without any risk to your health or wellbeing, in fact, quite the opposite. I've compiled this workbook full of action steps for you, with tips that have helped both me and my clients to learn to eat instinctively, to live a vibrant life and to feel well enough to enjoy everything it has to offer.

A GIFT FROM MY ANCESTORS

My nutrition coaching practice has also been through a transformative journey in many ways. I have tried, tested and experimented with all kinds of different ways to find what I believe is the key to helping others and myself. Funnily enough, while I was reading and studying the latest research, I realised the answer is much less complicated. Around that time I was struck with the simplicity of my Mi'kmaq and Acadian ancestors. By looking back at the lives and diets of my ancestors I had another 'ah-ha' moment which has led me to the place I am now in my practice. Below is a symbol that represents The Mi'kmaq Medicine Wheel, which is the perfect symbol of all the principles that I have taken on board in my practice. The concept of Empowered Eating involves so much more than what we eat and how we eat it.

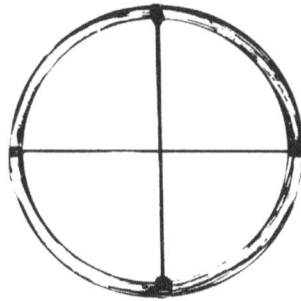

The Medicine Wheel is a circle divided into four equal parts. It is a ceremonial tool and the basis for all teaching wheels. In New Zealand, we have a similar representation for health, The Whare Tapa Wha created by Sir. Mason Durie. All over the world, many indigenous people share similar philosophies when it comes to health.

The power of the Four Directions is implied whenever a wheel or circle is drawn. Since traditional Native American cultures view life as a continuous cycle. Life mirrors the cycling of the seasons, the daily rising of the sun, and the phases of the moon. They also hold the view that all things are interrelated. The Medicine Wheel incorporates the powers of the Four Directions and the interrelatedness of all things.

The Medicine Wheel is also used as a teaching tool around what makes us healthy, happy humans and this is where I feel it powerfully represents the principles of my practice. I believe that if we can nourish all parts of the circle, we can experience health and happiness like never before.

The Medicine Wheel contains four key areas that need to be balanced to be our healthiest selves.

A GIFT FROM MY ANCESTORS

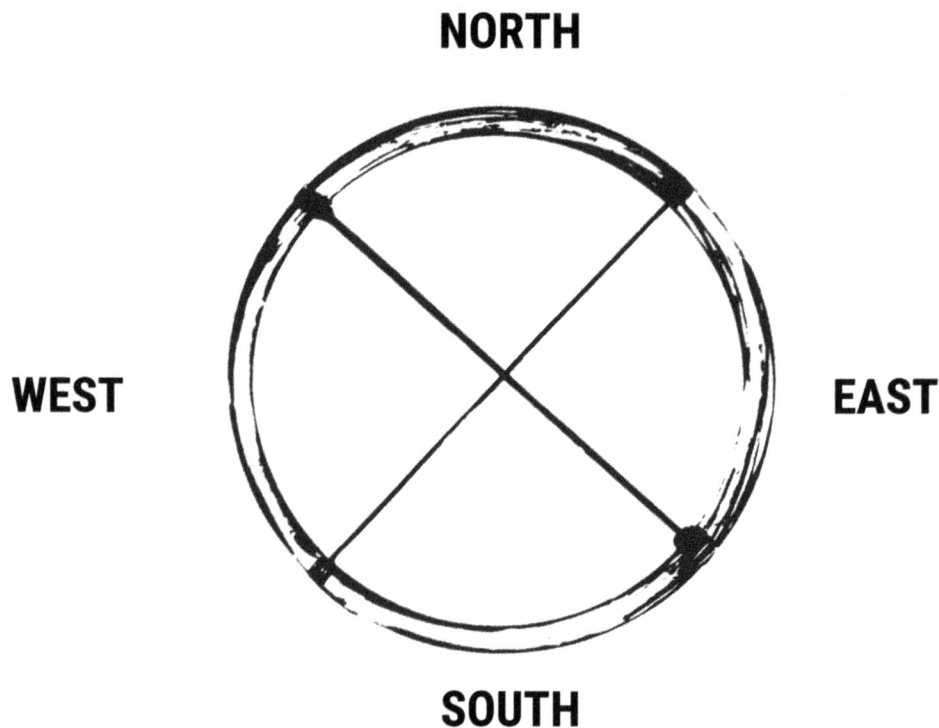

NORTH

WEST

EAST

SOUTH

The East represents the spiritual. For example, our relationship with nature, with our inner selves, with something higher than ourselves, and recognising synchronicity within the universe.

The South represents the emotional. This includes a positive self-image, -positive self-esteem, self-love, self-care, connection and a positive environment.

The West represents the physical. It includes a balanced diet, movement, sleep, stress management etc.

The North describes the cognitive or mental. This is all about keeping our mind stimulated and taking care of our mental wellbeing, whatever that looks like for each individual.

Should one of the four areas be missing or in some way damaged, a person or a collective may become 'unbalanced' and subsequently unwell. This is the cornerstone of Empowered Eating. The HUB of the wheel so to speak. If any of the areas are out of balance - they can also impact our relationship with food and our overall health.

WHAT IS EMPOWERED EATING?

Learning to listen to and trust your body again.

During the first year in my practice, I realised that there was a huge gap in my services and programs. Clients were coming to see me and losing heaps of weight, but they weren't keeping it off. This was followed many times by shame, which of course often resulted in them giving up altogether. My programs were giving people what they wanted short term, but were they really working if they didn't set you up for life? Absolutely not. In fact, they were doing the opposite, they were simply setting someone up for a lifetime of more ups and downs with the diet industry under the veil of "healthy eating". It was difficult for me when I realised this. Do I do what the industry does and blame the person because they couldn't do it? My conscience said no.

Later, after more digging and reading, I was determined to make some serious changes. I realised then that there is so much more to health than simply losing weight and just eating "real" food (whatever that means). In fact, weight loss and health do not always equate to the other. Taking care of our body is one thing but if we don't nourish the mind, heart and soul, we may continue to feel like food controls us.

Ultimately, if any part of the 'wheel' is out of balance, the rest will be as well. You can eat all the healthy foods in the world, but if you're stressed, it's not enough. If you are lonely and sad, eating well will also be difficult. If you are disconnected from your eating, you are likely to overeat and be left feeling uncomfortable... And the list goes on.

Through all this, the Medicine Wheel has been my anchor. It is now the cornerstone of all my teachings and programs and a permanent tattoo on my left wrist! So how does this relate to our eating habits? How does the Medicine Wheel teach us to feel empowered about our food choices? Let's explore each part.

Body:

In case you haven't noticed 'healthy eating' has become incredibly confusing! With Empowered Eating, nourishing our body is about turning our wisdom within and finding the foods that work best for our unique bodies. It's also about shifting our thinking from "I can't have this or that" to what foods you can add in that make you feel great. Interestingly, restricting certain foods is only going to make you want those foods even more. Ultimately, eating 'well' is about feeling well or at least, doing the best we can under our current circumstances.

WHAT IS EMPOWERED EATING?

It's also about finding ways to move your body in ways that you love rather than punishing yourself for that extra biscuit you had yesterday or to have six-pack abs. Movement can be functional (think gardening) or fun, and should not be the bane of your existence otherwise it's not enjoyable, and less likely to happen.

Nourishing our bodies is also about enjoying satisfying foods. Life is too short. If you don't enjoy it, don't eat it (whenever possible). We should never have to choke back healthy foods or diet drinks because someone told us to. There have even been studies that show that if we don't enjoy it, we don't absorb the nutrients as well anyways.

Nourishing your body is also about getting back into the kitchen and learning to prepare food for ourselves and our loved ones. Eating shouldn't be a chore it should be a gift that we offer our bodies with love and intention.

Heart:

The heart, our emotions. Have you ever eaten because you were sad, lonely or even bored? Identifying triggers is one of the cornerstones of Empowered Eating. It gives us an opportunity to feed the true need because if we're not hungry to begin with, no amount of food is going to satisfy us.

Empowered Eating is also about living your best life - whatever that looks like. Otherwise, we will crave food as a source of happiness (even if it is short term). That means taking care of yourself, setting boundaries, enjoying the outdoors, getting a haircut or a new pair of jeans and doing it now, not 5 kgs from now.

Connecting with each other and ourselves is also an important part of nourishing our hearts. Remembering to take time to connect with family, friends our community and acknowledging those who have come before us. And if this is difficult, it's about remembering to reach out and get the support you need.

When it comes to nourishing our hearts, it's also about compassion. Yes, we're going to have a bad day or week or even a bad year, but if we can be compassionate, it doesn't have to be the end of the road.

WHAT IS EMPOWERED EATING?

When it comes to the heart, Empowered Eating is a weight-neutral approach which means I'd love you to banish that scale once in for all. All the scale is going to do is weigh your self-worth and confidence and is not an accurate tool to measure our health.

Mind:

The mind is like the roots of a tree. Learning to listen to our body's wisdom, by engaging our mind, helps us feel empowered. Don't give up gluten just because someone on the internet told you to, especially if you can eat it and still feel amazing! Engage your mind, and your common sense.

Our mind is a crucial part of the wheel as well because our thoughts become our beliefs which then lead to actions. By engaging our mind we can be mindful of those thoughts around food, weight and ourselves that could be incorrect or holding us back.

Let's also engage our minds when it comes to appearance ideals. Did you know there was a time in history when you could buy cellulite cream to GIVE you cellulite? Times change, appearance ideals change, and they will continue to do so. Let your beauty be determined by those who love you and not some giant corporation that wants to earn a dollar (or a billion). Empowered Eating is about eating well because you want to take care of yourself and not because you think you should fit a particular mould, especially when the bar keeps changing.

We can also engage the mind and eat in an empowered way by bringing awareness into our eating. From awareness journals to pausing to ask if you're hungry to paying attention to our five senses when we engage in eating. Bringing consciousness into our eating habits is one of the most powerful tools you can use to break free from undesirable eating habits. By doing so, we will not only improve our digestion, but we can better identify triggers and learn to listen to and trust the innate wisdom of our bodies.

Empowered Eating is also about engaging your mind and paying attention to "head hunger". This is the hunger that comes when our bellies are full. If you're not hungry, no amount of food will satisfy and so by using our mind to identify head hunger vs real hunger we're better able to stop and ask ourselves if food is what we really need and guess what, sometimes, it's exactly what we need and that's ok too!

WHAT IS EMPOWERED EATING?

Spirit:

Nourishing our spirit does not have to be about prayer or religion (though those too can be powerful tools to help you on your journey). Engaging our spirit is about doing more of the things that make our soul sing but also about connecting with the people and the world around us. Our spirit is our purpose; it's what drives us, identify this, and you've got a powerful tool in overcoming disordered eating habits.

Nourishing our spirit is also about connecting. It's about saying thank you before meals and appreciating the journey that our food took to get to us and all the people, animals and plants involved. Lastly, it's about connecting to each other, putting down the cell phones, visiting instead of texting or emailing, holding hands, complementing one another supporting each other and caring about each other rather than comparing or putting each other down.

And so, while food is important, Empowered Eating is so much more than just what goes into our mouths; it's not just what we eat but how we eat and how we live. We can't have one without the other if we want to make peace with ourselves and the food we eat.

It's such a natural thing, our right as humans, but the most important part of Empowered Eating? It's taking things one step at a time and knowing that life is a roller coaster of fun and everything in between. To me, perfection is just recognising this and enjoying the ride while nourishing our body, mind, heart and spirit. We should never let perfection get in the way of this journey of learning and loving.

Within The Medicine Wheel, I have developed 8 principles of Empowered Eating. These principles create the backbone for a healthy relationship between food and ourselves.

1. Finding your 'why'
2. It's not your fault
3. Pressing pause
4. Tuning in
5. Fall in love with food again
6. Feed the need
7. Gentle nutrition
8. Live the life you crave

Ready to dig in?

THE EMPOWERED EATING PRINCIPLES

Find your 'why'

(1) Imagine starting on a journey with no map. You get kind of lost and take way longer to get to where you're going. So the first step of Empowered Eating is to taking time to focus on finding out what you really want! And when you've found out your destination we can create a really clear map of how to get there. Empowered Eating will help you find your 'why' and discover where you're going using proven strategies that unlock your inner motivations for long-lasting change.

It's not your fault

(2) Diet's suck. They just don't work. And it's got nothing to do with your lack of willpower or 'uncontrollable' cravings. Diets simply don't work long term. If they did you wouldn't be on your third, fourth or fifteenth one! Not only do diet not work but the whole process of dieting can be bad for you both mentally AND physically. Empowered Eating will teach you why they don't work and show you a better plan to achieve long term health.

Pressing pause

(3) Pressing pause is about stopping before eating to ask yourself if you really are hungry and if not, what it is that you actually need. Empowered Eating will show you how to listen to and honour your body's natural cues so you can eat for not just nourishment but energy and enjoyment as well! Setting the stage for rebuilding trust with food and yourself. And make decision of when and what to eat more of a conscious act.

THE EMPOWERED EATING PRINCIPLES

Tune in

4

There's power in paying attention to the act of eating. Eating mindfully, slowing down, enjoying our food, feeling fullness and making eating something to enjoy. Tuning in is about giving you the tools to listen to what your body needs as well as increasing the pleasure and satisfaction of eating! Empowered Eating will help you listen to how your body feels after eating, and experimenting with curiosity rather than rigid rules. So you can feel great before and after eating.

Fall in love with food again

5

All foods can be part of a healthy way of eating. But the restrictions we often put on our eating can lead to binges and feelings of being out of control. Leaving us feeling guilt, shame and so desperate to count points again. Together, through Empowered Eating, we'll show you how to begin to eat fearlessly again and let go of food rules so that you can feel great AND eat cake (or whatever else you love).

Feed the need/Rebuild the trust

6

If you're not hungry to begin with, no amount of food will fill you up. Learn to make peace with your emotions (without eating them!). Emotional eating can be a great clue that something's amiss. Together, at Empowered Eating, you'll learn how to tune into what's really going on so that you can start to feed the real need and stop the 'binge-repent-repeat' cycle in its tracks. Giving you alternative ways to comfort and care for yourself without food.

THE EMPOWERED EATING PRINCIPLES

Gentle nutrition

(7) After years of following diets, it's no wonder we're stuck in nutrition confusion. Nourishing our body is important and honouring it is one of many great tools for self-care. But what we choose to eat has got tangled up in what we 'can't' have or 'shouldn't have. Empowered Eating will help you clear up the nutrition confusion and help you choose more of the foods that make you feel great.

Live the life you crave

(8) The more we engage in the things that bring us joy and move our body in ways that feel good the less control food will have over us. Empowered Eating shows you a different way to break the diet cycle. Releasing you from obsessive thoughts about food so you can free up the mental space for what really makes you happy. It's time to feel comfortable in your own body, knowing you're respecting, nourishing, and taking care of yourself.

EATING PATTERNS QUESTIONNAIRE

This quiz will assess where you are on the intuitive eating scale. It can be a good way to measure the outcomes of this programme or just to gain some insight. It is adapted from Tracy Tylka's research on Tribole & Resch's model of Intuitive Eating (1,2,3]. This updated assessment was validated for use with both men and women and includes a new category, Body-Food Choice Congruence, which reflects Principle 10 of Intuitive Eating: Honour your health with gentle nutrition.

Directions: The following statements are grouped into the three core characteristics of intuitive eaters. Answer "yes" or "no" for each statement. If you are unsure of how to respond, consider if the description usually applies to you—is it mostly "yes" or "no"?

────────────────

SECTION 1: UNCONDITIONAL PERMISSION TO EAT

1. I try to avoid certain foods high in fat, carbs or calories: YES/ NO

2. If I am craving a certain food, I don't allow myself to have it: YES/ NO

3. I get mad at myself for eating something unhealthy: YES/ NO

4. I have forbidden foods that I don't allow myself to eat: YES/ NO

5. I don't allow myself to eat what food I desire at the moment: YES/ NO

6. I follow eating rules or diet plans that dictate what, when and/or how to eat: YES/NO

SECTION 2: EATING FOR EMOTIONAL RATHER THAN PHYSICAL REASONS

1. I find myself eating when I'm feeling emotional (anxious, sad, depressed), even when I'm not physically hungry: YES/ NO

2. I find myself eating when I am lonely, even when I'm not physically hungry: YES/ NO

3. I use food to help me soothe my negative emotions: YES/ NO

EATING PATTERNS QUESTIONNAIRE

4. I find myself eating when I am stressed out, even when I'm not physically hungry: YES/ NO

5. I am able to cope with my negative emotions (i.e. anxiety and sadness) without turning to food for comfort: YES/ NO

SECTION 3: RELIANCE ON INTERNAL HUNGER/SATIETY CUES (BODY TRUST)

1. I trust my body to tell me when to eat: YES/ NO

2. I trust my body to tell me what to eat: YES/ NO

3. I trust my body to tell me how much to eat: YES/ NO

4. I rely on my hunger signals to tell me when to eat: YES/ NO

5. I rely on my fullness (satiety) signals to tell me when to stop eating: YES/ NO

6. I trust my body when to stop eating: YES/ NO

SECTION 4: BODY-FOOD CHOICE CONGRUENCE

1. Most of the time, I desire to eat nutritious foods: YES/ NO

2. I mostly eat foods that make my body perform efficiently (well): YES/ NO

3. I mostly eat foods that give my body energy and stamina: YES/ NO

SCORING
• Sections 1-2: Each "yes" statement indicates an area that likely needs some work.
• Section 3-4: Each "no" statement indicates an area that likely needs some work.

MY SCORE:

Section 1: _____ Section 2: _____ Section 3: _____ Section 4: _____

Source
[1]. Tylka, Tracy L. (2006). Development and psychometric evaluation of a measure of intuitive eating. Journal of Counseling Psychology 53(2), Apr:226-240.
[2] Tylka, T.L. (2013). A psychometric evaluation of the Intuitive Eating Scale with college men.Journal of Counseling Psychology, Jan;60(1):137-53.
[3] Tribole E. & Resch E. (2012). Intuitive Eating (3rd ed). St.Martin's Press, NY:NY.

PRINCIPLE 1

FINDING YOUR WHY

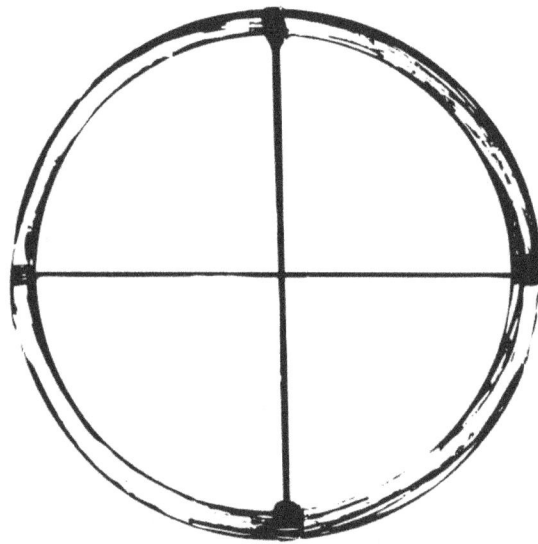

Imagine starting on a journey with no map. You get kind of lost and take way longer to get to where you're going. So the first step of Empowered Eating is to taking time to focus on finding out what you really want! And when you've found out your destination we can create a really clear map of how to get there. Empowered Eating will help you find your 'why' and discover where you're going using proven strategies that unlock your inner motivations for long-lasting change.

SETTING GOALS AND FINDING YOUR "WHY"

1. Start by thinking about what YOU really want. Not something you feel you 'should' do or because someone has told you to, this has to come from YOU for it to happen. Be clear, what is it that you really want? One of the biggest reasons people don't get what they want is because they don't actually know what it is that they want. Be specific. Do you want to be more energised? Do you want to stop the yo-yo diet cycle? Do you actually want to lose weight or it that you want more confidence?

_____

_____

_____

_____

_____

_____

2. Why do you want it? Sounds simple, but have a good think about your reasons or motivations because this is what will drive your heart, soul and ultimately your body, to get it done. How will life change once you achieve your goal?

_____

_____

_____

_____

_____

_____

3. How will I be different once I achieve these goals? What will life look like?

_____

_____

_____

_____

_____

_____

SETTING GOALS AND FINDING YOUR "WHY"

4. Why don't you have these goals already? A tricky question I know, but I want you to think about what mental or physical blocks are currently in place that are preventing you from achieving your goals. After all, if you've been stuck in a rut for a while now, something is obviously getting in the way. Maybe it's lack of clarity or something more physical? What are the barriers preventing you from realising your dreams? Figure this out and you're nearly there.

_____
_____
_____
_____
_____
_____

5. What is the **easiest** thing you can do to move in the right direction? Maybe it's simply engaging in this course 100% or maybe it's simply drinking more water. What's one thing you can focus your attention on, right now, to achieve your goals and change your life? Just one step is all you need.

_____
_____
_____
_____
_____
_____

SETTING S.M.A.R.T GOALS

When you set 'doable' goals, you'll achieve them more often. Goals provide focus, enhance productivity, boost self-esteem, and increase commitment. When setting a goal, clearly outline the steps needed to achieve it while minimizing overwhelm. Make your goals S.M.A.R.T. – Specific, Measurable, Attainable, Realistic, and Timely. With practice, you'll find that you're able to achieve more than you thought you could.

IS THE GOAL SPECIFIC?	IS THE GOAL MEASURABLE?	IS THE GOAL ATTAINABLE?	IS THE GOAL REALISTIC?	IS THE TIMING RIGHT?
Be as detailed as possible. The more specific you are, the more likely you are to reach the goal. For example: Want to work out more? What does that look like? 3 times a week? 4? Who would you go with? Will you get a trainer?	Establish criteria to measure progress. How will you know when the goal is achieved? Create a checklist of steps and check off each item as it's completed.	When you clearly identify your goal, you can embody the attitudes, abilities, and skills to reach it successfully. We often get caught up in what we think we should be doing instead of going after our core desires. Make sure your goals align with your future vision and authentic self.	You must be willing and able to work toward your goal. How committed are you? Be honest with yourself about your available time and energy and plan accordingly.	Anchor your goal with a deadline and create a calendar leading up to it with all the steps you need to take to reach your goal mapped out.

THE AWARENESS JOURNAL

Keeping a food diary can be a valuable tool for pushing the pause button and learning what drives your hunger. It can also be quite triggering for some and so take some time to check in to see if it will be of benefit. A food diary is not about counting your carbs or how many grammes of salmon you had. What I am asking is that you begin to notice when what and why you are eating certain things. It's not about counting calories – it's about creating consciousness.

A food diary is a record of what you are eating, where you ate it, how you ate, what time you ate and what thoughts and feelings surrounded that eating. The focus isn't on the foods as much as the feelings surrounding them and the amount of food that these feelings cause you to eat. It allows us to bring consciousness to our eating which is a powerful tool to be able to listen to our bodies again.

Ultimately, you can only change what you're aware of, so an awareness journal will be a place to record your observations about WHY, WHEN, WHAT, HOW, HOW MUCH you eat as well as WHERE you invest your energy.

Your diary could include the following:

• Time, day, where the food was consumed.

• What was my hunger level before?

• What was consumed? (Don't worry about calories or macros, just get a rough idea of what it was that you ate)

• Did I overeat? Did I undereat?

• Mindful eating scale (mark it 1-10). Did you eat the food in a rushed state (1) or take the time to eat mindfully and intentionally (10)?

• Feelings and thoughts

• Any triggers identified

You can use your own template - or one of the templates on the following pages. I've included additional sheets in the appendix of this workbook. Remember, a food diary such as this is about consciousness and curiosity and should never allow for guilt or shame for any food choices. We'll work through that together!

EMPOWERED EATING

Awareness
JOURNAL

Goals:

From _____ to _____

date/time	what	where	hunger level	mindful scale	triggers/thoughts

notes

Day 1

VEGGIES AND FRUIT	PROTEIN SOURCES

HEALTHY FATS	FIBRE SOURCES

CARB SOURCES	FERMENTED FOODS

ONE ACT OF SELF CARE

TODAY I AM GRATEFUL FOR

Day 2

VEGGIES AND FRUIT	PROTEIN SOURCES

HEALTHY FATS	FIBRE SOURCES

CARB SOURCES	FERMENTED FOODS

ONE ACT OF SELF CARE

TODAY I AM GRATEFUL FOR

LEARNING FROM YOUR AWARENESS JOURNAL

If you've decided to complete an awareness journal or food diary you can begin to use that information to make some powerful observations. There are several questions that can help us to gather useful information about any undesired behaviours or patterns. Analysing your journal will add in 'next level' consciousness when it comes to eating.

- Are there certain foods that trigger more eating?
- What times do you eat? Do you sometimes go long periods without eating anything at all? Why?
- Are periods of restrictive eating sometimes followed by binging?
- Are there places or times that seem to be conducive to overeating?
- What do you notice about the times you eat?
- What is fuelling your need to feed when you're not hungry?
- Do you eat because of emotions? Which ones?
- Are your meal times working for you?
- What other patterns do you notice when it comes to your eating behaviour?

Use the questions above to begin to observe patterns and behaviours around food. Begin to come up with some loving behaviours that you want to implement in the week ahead. Use the space below to jot down any thoughts or ideas.

SMALL STEPS

Let's get this out of the way right now, before we even get too far into the programme. If you've ever been on a diet (as most of us have) you know their approach is all or nothing. But the problem with 'all or nothing' is exactly that. You're either doing it all or nothing at all and neither has led to long term health outcomes or peace of mind right? We can also find ourselves feeling guilty if we don't give it 100%

So, if you're feeling a bit unmotivated or discouraged at any point in this programme, I would like to remind you that this program is not about a complete overhaul overnight because as we've learned that doing this often does not work in the long term. On the other hand, small meaningful steps will lead to lasting behaviour change. We will cover A LOT of material and many of it will be very new. Be kind to yourself and start with what resonates with you.

Just take one step, just one. Master that step, find your stride, and once that is part of everyday life take another one.

A complete overhaul doesn't provide the change you're after long term, but mastering each step you take will certainly get you closer to your goals. It may seem to take longer but how long has it taken you to get to this point where enough is enough? And so, if you only did one thing from this program. Just one step. You'll still be heading in the right direction.

If you feel like you've 'fallen off the wagon' or that you are not making progress, perhaps you've taken on too much, maybe you're comparing this to diets you've done, or maybe it's time to put the scale away once and for all. Be compassionate with yourself and potentially scale things back a bit.

"Do what you can with what you have, where you are"
- Theodore Roosevelt

BLACK AND WHITE THINKING

We all have thoughts. Some are helpful and some are not. By being aware of our thoughts and identifying which are true or not as well as which to engage with we can begin to have a more positive relationship with food and our bodies.

One very common thought pattern in regards to eating is known as 'black and white thinking'. We do A LOT of black and white thinking when it comes to food.

When someone is engaging in black and white thinking they will label certain foods as "good" or "bad", "healthy" or "naughty", "clean or "junk food" and usually feel guilty or anxious if they eat something that they consider to be wrong or bad. Black and white thinking can sound like:

- I feel like eating chocolate, but I'll have some 'nice cream' instead.
- II can eat this but if I do, I'm going to have to work it off tomorrow
- I blew it today, that's ok, I'll start on my diet tomorrow.
- I already ate a cookie today, I've blown, I might as well keep going

This back and forth thinking can be really friggen exhausting emotionally! Have you ever had thoughts like this in regards to food? If you're like me, I'm sure you've thought this way at some point in your life.

But how does labelling foods in this way influence our eating patterns? Does it influence your enjoyment of the food? I'd say 'absolutely right?

But what happens when we mix black and white together. What colour do we get? Grey. Ah… I love this grey area! Maybe if we listened to our bodies AND our brains our thoughts would be a bit more balanced. It might sound a little like this:

- I kind of want something crunchy and salty. I think I'll have some carrots and some chips.
- Pizza sounds good, but I'm craving veggies too. I think I'll have a salad with my pizza.
- I feel like being active, but I don't feel like running today. I think I'll go for a walk.

BLACK AND WHITE THINKING

Consider a yo-yo. Well just like yo-yo dieting yo-yos go up and down and so do our thoughts and our body weight when we diet. Our thoughts and weight is either UP or down, right? It doesn't usually stop n the middle.

However, if we drop it right down it might just start to swing a bit, side to side like a pendulum.

When we label foods 'bad' and restrict those foods the yo-yo gets pulled all the way to one side and we can stay here, restricting, eating keto bars, pretending paleo bread tastes just like regular bread. Until one night, you're out to dinner and the waiter shows up with the breadbasket. Eventually, we give in right? And so what happens to the yo-yo? It then swings all the way to the other side.

This is our internal voice that says 'stuff this' I'm eating the whole f'ing basket of bread. I've already ruined it, I might as well keep going. Not only that but when I'm home tonight I'm going to pick up a tub of two of ice cream to top it off. It's ok, I'll just get back to it tomorrow. Then we feel guilty and we do start again tomorrow. Making the yo-yo go back and forth back and forth... for years and years. It's either all or nothing right?

But what if we don't go this far over to the restricting side? We see then that we don't go so far over to the overdoing it side. Eventually, we will find this nice happy middle ground.

Because if you stop pulling the yo-yo, hop off the yo-yo dieting cycle, eventually it will stop swinging.

Maybe not straight away, it will take time to lose momentum just like it takes a while to get rid of that diet mentality. But that's what Empowered Eating sets out to do. To help us find this nice little middle ground with a healthy relationship with food without losing our shit. It's possible I promise you!

THE FLYING TRAPEZE

Sometimes, I feel that my life is a series of trapeze swings. I'm either hanging on to a trapeze bar swinging along or, for a few moments, I'm hurdling across space between the trapeze bars.

Mostly, I spend my time hanging on for dear life to the trapeze bar of the moment. It carries me along a certain steady rate of swing and I have the feeling that I'm in control. I know most of the right questions, and even some of the right answers. But once in a while, as I'm merrily, or not so merrily, swinging along, I look ahead of me into the distance, and what do I see?

I see another trapeze bar looking at me. It's empty. And I know, in that place in me that knows, that this new bar has my name on it. It is my next step, my growth, my aliveness coming to get me. In my heart of hearts I know that for me to grow, I must release my grip on the present well-known bar to move to the new one.

Each time it happens, I hope—no, I pray—that I won't have to grab the new one. But in my knowing place, I know that I must totally release my grasp on my old bar, and for some moments in time I must hurtle across space before I can grab the new bar. Each time I do this I am filled with terror. It doesn't matter that in all my previous hurdles I have always made it.

Each time I am afraid I will miss, that I will be crushed on unseen rocks in the bottomless basin between the bars. But I do it anyway. I must. Perhaps this is the essence of what the mystics call faith. No guarantees, no net, no insurance, but we do it anyway because hanging on to that old bar is no longer an option. And so, for what seems to be an eternity but actually lasts a microsecond. I soar across the dark void called "the past is over, the future is not yet here." It's called a transition. I have come to believe that it is the only place that real change occurs.

I have a sneaking suspicion that the transition zone is the only real thing, and the bars are the illusions we dream up to not notice the void. Yes, with all the fear that can accompany transitions, they are still the most vibrant, growth-filled, passionate moments in our lives. And so transformation of fear may have nothing to do with making fear go away, but rather with giving ourselves permission to "hang out" in the transition zone -- between the trapeze bars -- allowing ourselves to dwell in the only place where change really happens.

It can be terrifying. It can also be enlightening. Hurdling through the void, we just may learn to fly.

Excerpted from Warriors of the Heart by Danaan Perry.

MY NOTES

MY NOTES

PRINCIPLE 2

IT'S NOT YOUR FAULT

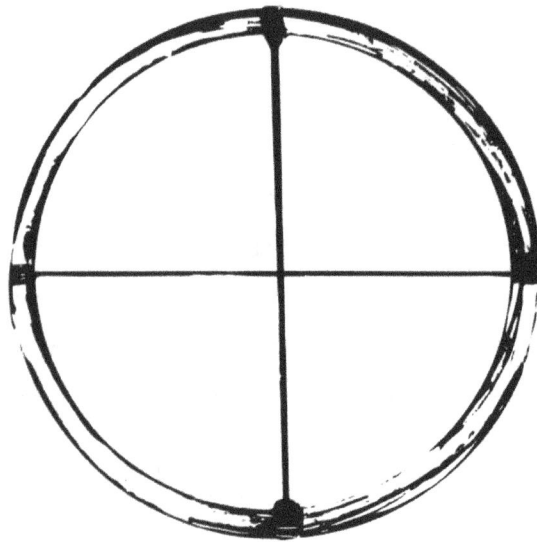

Diet's suck. They just don't work. And it's got nothing to do with your lack of willpower or 'uncontrollable' cravings. Diets simply don't work long term. If they did you wouldn't be on your third, fourth or fifteenth one! Not only do diets not work but the whole process of dieting can be bad for you both mentally AND physically. Empowered Eating will teach you why they don't work and show you a better plan to being a healthier version of you.

IT'S NOT YOUR FAULT...

RAISE YOUR HAND IF YOU'VE EVER BEEN ON A DIET.

You'll often hear us talking about "diets" and you're probably envisioning Jenny Craig, Weight Watchers, Noom, Slimming World etc.

Diets, unfortunately, are much more common than that. A lot of various eating plans out there are often diets in disguise. So what is a diet and how can you tell the difference? There are some red flags to keep an eye out for:

• The ultimate goal is weight loss and is the predominant measure of success.
• You feel guilt or shame if you eat something 'unhealthy' or 'off the plan'.
• You have less energy on this way of eating.
• You feel anxious about eating at social events.
• You don't feel confident to know what to eat or cook without the 'plan'?
• You have rules that you need to follow (no bread? No ice cream? etc.)
• You are often hungry and/or thinking about food.
• You have to count calories, macros and/or points
• You feel restricted in any way.
• You can't have your favourite food unless it's a 'cheat day'

If you've answered yes to any of these questions, chances are your healthy eating plan is just another diet and no, it's not a 'lifestyle' if it's unsustainable and sucks the fun out of food. A healthy eating plan involves a healthy mindset and later we'll spend some time identifying why. For now, just know that any way of eating that encourages you to ditch your favourite foods completely (unless you need to for medical reasons) is unfortunately just a diet. The bottom line is – they are not sustainable, and if it's not sustainable the effects can sometimes be worse for our health than the so-called 'evil' foods you were giving up in the first place.

So, if you've been there, done that, dieted and dieted again and the weight just won't stay off, you're binging, you're giving up, or any of the above. I want you to know 4 words:

It's NOT your fault.

Seriously, diets don't work. In 60%- 97% of all cases, diets are only a short-term fix with the weight loss inevitably being regained (and then some). A prominent medical journal stated "in controlled settings, participants who remain in weight loss programmes usually lose 10% of their weight. However, half to two-thirds of the weight is regained within one year, and almost all is regained within 5 years. If you've been on a diet before, or several diets, you've likely experienced this first hand.

Diets can also have serious physical and psychological consequences and yet we find ourselves trapped in a never-ending vicious cycle of yo-yo dieting.

THE DIETING CYCLE

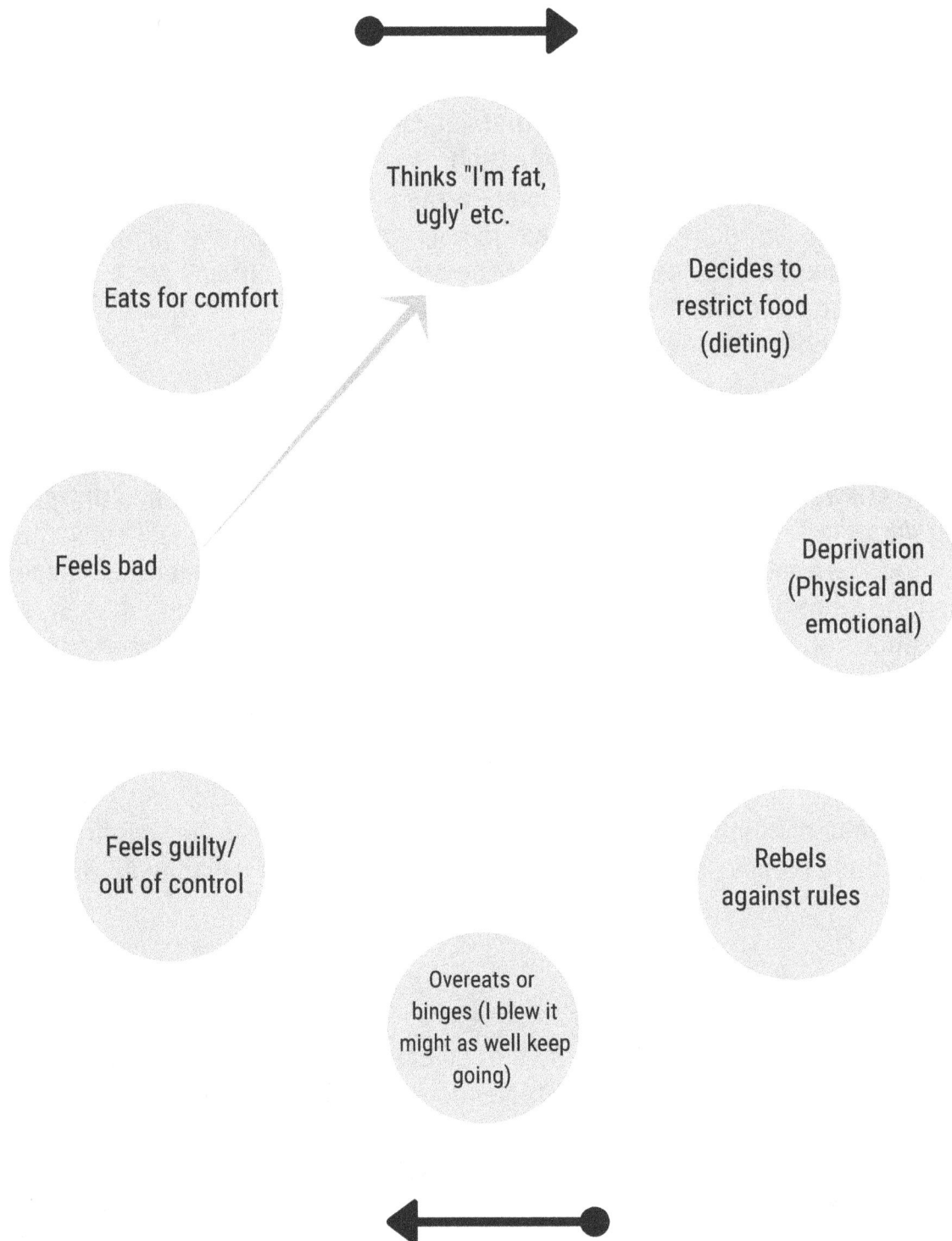

Thinks "I'm fat, ugly' etc.

Decides to restrict food (dieting)

Eats for comfort

Deprivation (Physical and emotional)

Feels bad

Rebels against rules

Feels guilty/ out of control

Overeats or binges (I blew it might as well keep going)

IT'S NOT YOUR FAULT...

DOES THIS CYCLE SOUND FAMILIAR?

This continuing vortex is known as "diet culture" and it is a difficult ride to hop off of. For some, this can go on for years even decades. It's not your fault, and that's why we're here.

The cycle can continue in different places, but almost always starts with the decision to diet. Why not? We feel in control, even if it is for just a short time. It's the consequences that leave us feeling miserable though through both physical and emotional deprivation.

I highly recommend you watch the TED talk by **Sandra Aamodt: "Why dieting doesn't usually work**" which goes deeper into her own personal story as well as an introduction to Set Point Theory. You can also learn more from Lindo Bacon in her book "Health at Every Size©" and "Body Respect". I highly recommend you do so.

BUT WHAT ABOUT HEALTH?

You may be wondering, "what if I need to lose weight because I want to prevent disease or I want to manage a condition that I already have?"

There's nothing wrong with wanting to feel well and comfortable– the myth is that weight is the cause of all the disease or pain in the world.

It's true that there is a correlation between excess weight and disease (though not in all cases). But as you may have heard many many times. Correlation does not mean causation. That would be like saying that yellow teeth give us lung cancer because so many people with yellow teeth get lung cancer. In fact, it's cigarette smoking that is the biggest cause amongst other things including genetics.

Think about this question – if someone has really unhealthy habits, is stressed, not sleeping but is skinny are they guaranteed not to get diabetes, sore joints, cancer etc? Or in another case imagine someone who eats incredibly well, is happy and moves their body regularly but is in a bigger body are they actually 'unhealthy'? Health is not determined by weight, full stop.

IT'S NOT YOUR FAULT...

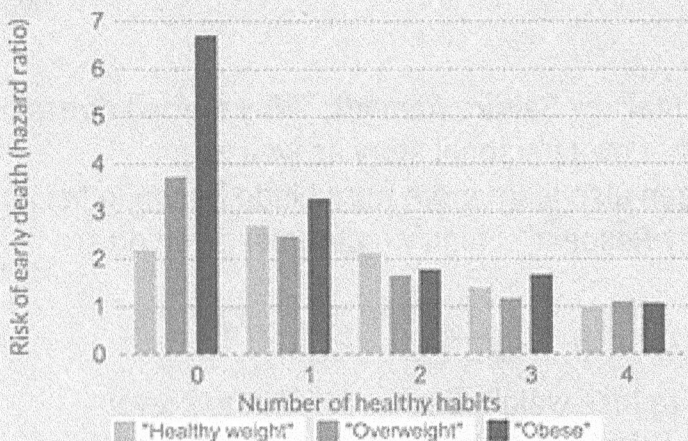

HEALTHY HABITS

www.healthnatdiets.com

Risk of dying early is influenced more by behaviours than by weight

Risk of early death (hazard ratio)

Number of healthy habits

■ "Healthy weight"   ■ "Overweight"   ■ "Obese"

Matheson, Eric M., Dana E. King, and Charles J. Everett. "Healthy lifestyle habits and mortality in overweight and obese individuals." The Journal of the American Board of Family Medicine 25.1 (2012): 9-15.

Healthy habits that count:

Eat five or more fruit &/or vegetables each day

Get some exercise more than 12 times a month

Drink a little alcohol (up to 1 drink for women and 2 for men each day)

Don't smoke

By changing our habits to those that nurture and care for our bodies, we are increasing our life expectancy, our energy and motivation improves and our overall well being is improved. This happens regardless of weight loss. I'm not saying that healthy habits won't result in weight loss in some cases but each experience is different and regardless of weight loss, health is improved significantly.

There are plenty of unwell skinny people and plenty of people who are in bigger bodies that are healthy and vibrant. Health does not discriminate like we do.

Let's instead focus on health as a feeling – not a look – and once we can do that. That is when the magic happens.

Are you ready to put that scale away (if you haven't yet) and break free from yo-yo dieting once and for all? Read on.

MY PAST DIETING STRATEGIES

We've been there done that! Diets make a lot of promises - but do they keep them?
List all the dieting programs you have tried in the past to lose weight or change your
shape. What were the results? Why do you think they didn't work long term?

What I've tried	Results	Why it didn't work

HOW HAS DIETING INTERFERED WITH YOUR LIFE?

Directions: This list includes consequences that result from dieting (note this is not all-inclusive). Check all that apply to you

Physical

Do you have signs of?

- [ ] Weight gain
- [ ] Blunted metabolism
- [ ] Cravings for carbs
- [ ] Blood sugar swings
- [ ] Disconnect from hunger cues
- [ ] Disconnect from satiety cues
- [ ] Chronically tired, even when sleeping well
- [ ] Hair falling out
- [ ] Inconsistent menses
- [ ] Feeling 'numb' physically
- [ ] Other _____

Social

When people are present do you _?

- [ ] I eat differently
- [ ] I compare my food to what others are eating
- [ ] I worry what others think about my eating.
- [ ] I worry about what people think about my body
- [ ] I try to eat the same type and quantity of food that others are eating
- [ ] I cancel social events because of the food served
- [ ] I avoid eating
- [ ] My behaviours and beliefs about my eating and body have interfered with relationships
- [ ] Other _____

Psychological

Do you have moods or thoughts of _?

- [ ] I worry about my eating
- [ ] I have strict rules about eating
- [ ] I count calories, carbs or other.
- [ ] Good vs bad food thinking
- [ ] I feel guilty when I eat bad food
- [ ] Mood swings
- [ ] I am afraid of feeling hungry
- [ ] I am afraid of feeling too full.
- [ ] I don't trust my body
- [ ] I'm afraid to eat 'forbidden food'.
- [ ] I am pre-occupied by thoughts of what I eat and don't eat.
- [ ] Fantasise about food
- [ ] Other _____

Behaviour

Do you engage in this behaviour?

- [ ] If I break a food rule, I eat even more of it.
- [ ] If I eat too much, I make up for it by skipping a meal or eating less food, even if I'm hungry.
- [ ] I eat more food when I'm stressed.
- [ ] I exercise only to burn calories or lose weight
- [ ] I talk a lot about dieting, weight and food.
- [ ] When I'm on vacation I ignore my food rules and eat whatever I want no matter how full I feel.
- [ ] Binge eating
- [ ] Avoiding physical intimacy
- [ ] Other _____

HEALTH AND WEIGHT

If you are feeling uncomfortable in your body because you've put on weight, it's understandable that you would want to change your body, we've got a whole heap of pressure from everyone around us to do so. But, it's important to know that it's the healthy behaviours that improve our health. Weight loss is not a behaviour.

Instead, if we can work out WHY we're having difficulty achieving health, make individual, and sustainable behavioural changes, we're more likely to achieve long-term health benefits.

There are several other reasons why we should avoid the number on the scale when it comes to setting long-term goals.

1. Often, our weight loss goals are set against unrealistic standards. They are based on the current culture's appearance ideals and not what might be healthiest for that individual. An individual's healthy weight is different to another just like a shoe size. When someone adapts healthy habits and takes care of themselves on a daily basis, their bodies may then go to a naturally healthy state - for them.

2. A healthy weight can change for an individual over time. It's difficult to achieve a goal weight that we can maintain as our body changes.

3. Focusing on the scale, or counting calories takes away our innate ability to listen to our own bodies cues. It is not reflective of any positive changes in behaviours.

4. Your weight does not define you or make you more or less valuable as a person. Bodies are beautiful, diverse and constantly evolving. What message do you want to teach the children in your life?

You are worth more than that number!

THE WEIGHT OF THE SCALE

How do you feel about not weighing yourself for the remainder of this program? What emotions come up for you?

_____
_____
_____
_____
_____

2. Does this make you feel anxious? Why? What would happen if you didn't weigh yourself?

_____
_____
_____
_____
_____

3. What other ways could you measure health?

_____
_____
_____
_____
_____

BANISH APPEARANCE IDEALS

As I've said before, there are many factors that influence what we believe our healthy weight is. Funnily enough, none of them seem to revolve around how we're feeling and health in general. Nope, what appears to influence what we believe our healthy weight should be is determined by several external societal factors. Ugh.

- Where you live.
- Someone else's opinion (doctors, friends, families, bloggers)
- The media
- What decade you live in.
- Your race

And I'm sure there are heaps more...

These are called appearance ideals and guess what. They change, all the time.

We've gone from "Gilmore Girls" to "waifs" to "Bootylicious" over the past 60 years and everything in between. In the times of Marylyn Munroe it was an era of "bring on those curves!" and in 10 years from now, some other body size will be the pot of gold at the end of the rainbow. Ultimately, the bar keeps changing.

There is good evidence to suggest that fatphobia has racial origins as well. I highly recommend the book "Fearing the Black Body" by Sabrina Springs as well as The Body Is Not An Apology" by Sonia Renee Taylor for more info on this.

Sizes and appearances, in general, go in and out of fashion (thank goodness for that because my hair in the eighties is something that need never return!).

For most of us here in New Zealand, the ideal body size that is portrayed in the media is one that is, for women, around 178cm weighing roughly 60 kilos However, the average New Zealand woman weighs about 72.6 kg and is 164cm tall.

There are so many different shapes, heights and weights for women all over the world and yet we continue to compare ourselves to standards that portray less than 10% of all women. It's an unachievable goal that is making the dieting industry rich and us miserable.

BANISH APPEARANCE IDEALS

These strict appearance ideals increase body dissatisfaction and can lead to eating disorders, yo-yo dieting and all around problematic relationships with food, exercise and each other.

The message here is to try to accept beauty as individual and better yet, to redefine beauty. Our bodies are a gift from the long line of ancestors before us.

Appearance ideals change and they will continue to do so. Respect yourself in your natural beauty and strive to feel amazing physically and mentally so that you can do all the amazing things that your body is meant to do.

"Now every girl is expected to have Caucasian blue eyes, full Spanish lips, a classic button nose, hairless Asian skin with a California tan, a Jamaican dance hall ass, long Swedish legs, small Japanese feet, the abs of a lesbian gym owner, the hips of a nine-year-old boy, the arms of Michelle Obama, and doll tits."

- Tina Fey

MIDDLE AGE AND WEIGHT GAIN

As I'm writing this I'm 43, which for some would classify me as 'middle-age I guess, depending on how long I will live. As you would have seen in my story, while growing up I battled with my weight and body through yo-yo dieting and obsessing about the moral (health) value of food.

As I've gotten older, I have noticed that while nothing else has changed, my body was beginning to and for someone with a history of disordered eating – this was an incredibly triggering time for me. However, thankfully, over these past few years, I've learned a lot about health and that knowledge has helped me to maintain a healthy relationship with food despite being a bit heavier in the hips (and a few more greys and wrinkles!) My goal is that this course can help others to know that it's ok, that our bodies change, and that no matter what, we deserve to care for, nourish and respect our bodies – most definitely – without diets.

THE PROBLEM
When we think of disordered eating we often have visions of the young teenage emancipated (often white) woman. Coincidentally, the two times that disordered eating can peak for women are in those TWO big critical or sensitive periods of reproductive hormone change. Puberty was the most common time that we witness the start of dieting, restrictive behaviours and in some cases eating disorders, however, there is another overlooked critical hormonal change period that is often overlooked but just as dangerous a time for these behaviours – menopause.

Ah, just when we thought it couldn't get worse!

Although most cases still appear in adolescent girls and young women, an alarming shift has occurred. Eating disorders are now on the rise among middle-aged and older women as we see an increasing number of middle-aged women from highly industrialised countries are practising disordered eating behaviours.

I'd like to personally argue that these behaviours may not be so much 'on the rise' as they are now more openly talked about and studied. Regardless, we are hearing about more and more restrictive and disordered eating habits amongst middle-aged women. What do I mean by disordered eating? This can be a wide range of behaviours, that may not include diagnosed eating disorders anorexia or bulimia. Instead, it could look like excessive restrictive eating, yo-yo dieting etc, restrained eating in general, and an unhealthy obsession with food or body.

So why are we starting to see more and more middle-aged women battling with restrictive eating patterns and in some cases even full-blown eating disorders?

MIDDLE AGE AND WEIGHT GAIN

Put simply, the lower our self-esteem the more inclined we are to engage in disordered eating behaviours. And thanks to several factors to sway us this way, menopause can be the perfect storm for rigid restriction, disordered eating and full-blown eating disorders.

We've had a whole lifetime of diet dogma ingrained in our minds, perhaps we suffered from disordered eating or an eating disorder when we were younger, or maybe we have always had a stable weight but suddenly… our hip/belly size seems to be increasing. This can be scary and frustrating for women and there are many reasons why we might suddenly start to engage in unhealthy restrictive behaviours during menopause. Two major ones include:

Our body changes: Let's make this 100% clear – it's NORMAL to put on extra weight, especially around your middle as our bodies age. This is often due to hormonal changes but can also be a result of doing less movement as we grow older. We know for many who have had a history of dieting and fighting this weight that this can be incredibly scary, especially in a society that demonises 'fatness'. Due to these hormonal shifts and excess weight gain we can easily start to relapse into our old or even very recent disordered eating habits. How much, or whether we gain weight at all is completely individual. But we need to accept the normality (and beauty) of the curves we develop as we grow older.

Being a middle-aged woman is hard work! Mid-life and beyond is often the time when major life events happen. Maybe you buy a home (or move into a better one), children move out, divorce, ageing parents, losing friends or family, stressful careers and let's not forget societal pressures to look like our 20-year-old selves! It would make sense that we would feel the need to control something when everything else is very much out of control, and difficult. Much like a teenager has their stresses, I'd like to say that the problems we face at mid-age are even more intense.

"It's a kind of cultural toxicity. We're told that to be seen, to get a promotion, to keep a romantic partner's interest, we have to be thin and trim. That pressure ends up being a far greater risk factor for disordered eating than are estrogen and serotonin sensitivity – and they affect a far greater number of women."
-Nutrition therapist and eating disorder specialist Julie Duffy Dillon

Because our bodies change – the societal pressures to look like our younger selves are bigger and worse than ever. It's a vicious cycle – our bodies naturally change thanks to hormones and other factors and yet the societal pressure is still there, if not increasing, to look a certain way.

MIDDLE AGE AND WEIGHT GAIN

In addition to this, us 'older' women are also more reluctant to seek help. We think we should 'just get over it' and dieting and restrictive eating behaviours are 'perfectly acceptable in a society that wants us to look younger. The urge is there to go back on diets, the stricter the better – anything to look like our 21-year-old self right? But, as we've said over and over again – the diets just don't work and it's a shift in mindset that is what is actually needed.

The problem with dieting and restrictive eating as a middle-aged woman is that weight cycling is harder on our bodies in general and especially as we age. The biggest cause of weight gain is the very thing we do to stop it – dieting. And the fluctuating changes to our weight over the years can have a variety of negative impacts on our health (and wellbeing).

Dieting itself can lead to further disordered eating – including overeating and binging.

"Dieting leads to bingeing. It's science. Say you skip breakfast to try and be 'good'. Your brain is pissed. It sends out neurotransmitters and hormones like ghrelin and neuropeptide Y – both of which are super potent orexigenic, meaning that they stimulate the appetite. So as the day goes on, these guys build-up, you give in (to your normal biological urge to eat) and once you pop you can't stop."

– London Institute for Intuitive Eating

Causes added stress (especially when they don't work) Damned if you do damned if you don't! Have you noticed that the more you diet, the harder the next diet is to maintain? They get harder to stay on.

Not only that, all this weight cycling, binging, and generally feeling out of control around food affects not only our metabolism but our self-esteem as well. This, we know is then coincided with disordered eating and so... the cycle continues. It is a pony ride we can't get off. Round and round we go.

This course/workbook will provide you with the steps to take to have a healthier relationship with your body and food. Go through the steps – reach out for support if needed. You've still got a whole heck of life to live.

WHAT IS ©HEALTH AT EVERY SIZE?

I want to introduce to you a health philosophy that may or may not be new to you. There are a lot of misconceptions about what ©HAES actually means which can lead to debates that aren't guided by facts. However, once most people read the key principles of ©HAES there's usually very little room for debate. So, what are the ©HAES principles?

1. **Weight Inclusivity:** Accept and respect the inherent diversity of body shapes and sizes and reject the idealizing or pathologizing of specific weights.

2. **Health Enhancement:** Support health policies that improve and equalize access to information and services, and personal practices that improve human well-being, including attention to individual physical, economic, social, spiritual, emotional, and other needs.

3. **Respectful Care:** Acknowledge our biases, and work to end weight discrimination, weight stigma, and weight bias. Provide information and services from an understanding that socio-economic status, race, gender, sexual orientation, age, and other identities impact weight stigma and support environments that address these inequities.

4. **Eating for Well-being**: Promote flexible, individualized eating based on hunger, satiety, nutritional needs, and pleasure, rather than any externally regulated eating plan focused on weight control.

5. **Life-Enhancing Movement:** Support physical activities that allow people of all sizes, abilities, and interests to engage in enjoyable movement, to the degree that they choose.

https://asdah.org/health-at-every-size-haes-approach/

Ultimately, HAES is simply the appreciation of size diversity, health-promoting behaviours and equal access to care and belonging for all individuals regardless of their body shape or size. I encourage you to read more about HAES© as it may be helpful for you to do so along this journey.

Have you ever experienced stigma from others, including medical professionals because of the size of your body?

_____

_____

CLEANSE YOUR NEWSFEED

This week I want you to start to pay close attention to your newsfeed, to marketing, to everything! Everywhere you look there are messages telling you that you are not enough, and that is how they make billions of dollars. You're not skinny enough; you're not healthy enough, you're not pretty enough, you're not fit enough.

They prey upon our vulnerability and your need to fit in and be accepted by the 'pack' and just keep chipping away at our very essence. To say it angers me would be an understatement because I too fell for it for far too long.

Take some time to analyse your newsfeed on social media. Are there messages that make you feel like you're not doing enough? That you're not enough because of your size or state of health? Begin to look at who is represented in your social media feed. What do the people you follow look like? Is there size diversity? Diversity of abilities? Gender diversity? Racial diversity? Or, is your newsfeed crowded with white skinny-fitspo or messages to 'quit this - quit that?' If so, it's time for a cleanse. Choose to 'unfollow' these pages and crowd in some of the inspirational and body-positive sites that I've listed below and on the next page instead.

This was a life-changing step in my own healing and many of the people I've worked with. I hope it helps you as well.

@everything_endocrine
@dont_fear_food
@meg.boggs
@shame.less.nutrition
@thebodypositive
@chronicwellnessnutrition
@missfitsworkout
@adolescent.nutritionist
@the_motivate_her
@fatdoctoruk
@notquitebeyonce
@wellseek
@edrdpro
@iamjesssanders

MORE INSTAGRAM PAGES TO FOLLOW

@michelle.m.yandle
@empowered_eating_coach
@nznutritionist
@lindobacon
@eatwellnz
@sweatypalsnz
@emmawrightbodyblossom
@mwnutr
@nude_nutritionist
@themindfuldietician
@moderationmovement
@feelgoodeating
@bethpilcherlisw
@bodypositive_mom
@damnthediets
@isarobinson_nutrition
@evelyntribole
@notplantbased
@fionawiller
@nanny_macb
@laurathomasphd
@pixienutrition
@no.food.rules
@marcird
@journey_to_wellness
@with_this_body
@theantidietplan
@girlsgonestrong
@emilyfonnesbeck_rd
@kristamuriascoach
@dieticiananna
@diets_dont_work_haes
@thenutritiontea
@melrobbins
@henrythecoloradodog (because cuteness)
@bodyposipanda
@sonyareneetaylor
@diabetes.rd

@mollyjforbes
@foodandfearless
@damnthediets
@louisegreen_bigfitgirl
@thebodylovesociety
@steph_gadreau
@black.nutritionist
@kids.nutritionist
@i_weigh
@lizzobeeating
@the_motivate_her
@chr1styharrison
@drjoshuawolrich
@secretlifeofemotionaleating
@bestsiide
@chantalcuthersnutritionist

Add your own:

NAVIGATING FEAR OF WEIGHT GAIN

So, you've embarked on this journey of Empowered Eating and it all sounds great and you feel great. You're loving the feeling of food freedom and the joy it brings to your life but then… You may start to reclaim weight that was lost from restrictive eating and this – well, can be terrifying for some. It would be unrealistic to think that you would suddenly start wholeheartedly loving your body after years of doing everything possible to change it. But, ultimately, when we embark on this journey towards empowered eating – We have no idea what our body will do.

Firstly, I want to acknowledge that this desire to lose weight is normal and understandable. We live in a fatphobic society that values and obsesses over thinness. We judge and feel judged. Sadly, fat people are often treated worse than thin people.

This fear comes from the false idea that each individual has the ability to control and manipulate their weight to a certain specific number or range. And further, that it's a person's responsibility to do so; and not doing or choosing not to is a personal failure. In reality, this is diet culture's failure, not yours.

"The weight loss industry is the only industry where a customer buys a product that doesn't work and the manufacturer blames the customer." – Evelyn Tribole

It's important to know that despite what we've been taught for probably our entire life, weight gain isn't necessarily unhealthy. If the habits we've implemented in the past have been rigid, restrictive etc then chances are weight gain is not something we need to worry about. We've already explained why weight doesn't equate health – but that doesn't get rid of the fear, I know.

Unfortunately, we can't wave a magic wand and simply wash these fears away and start loving our body as it is! Trust me, I understand. What we can do, however, is start the process towards accepting our body as it is, and wherever it is at its healthiest. Remember that health is more than just what we eat and how we look – it's a feeling and if feelings of anxiety, worry or fear revolving around food and our weight are present – this isn't living our healthiest life.

So how can we begin to decrease this fear around gaining weight? We're all different, but I will share some things that have helped me.

NAVIGATING FEAR OF WEIGHT GAIN

1. Begin by asking some questions and doing some reflection.

- Where did my fear of weight gain come from?
- Where are these messages coming from?
- Why do I value thinness?
- What is my opinion on those in larger bodies?
- Why do I think I am unlovable if my pant size increases?
- How are these opinions and beliefs impacting me? Are they in line with my values?
- What evidence do I have for or against these beliefs?
- How does weighing myself impact me?
- "What is this fear costing me in my school/work, relationships, health and happiness?"
- If I don't let go of this fear, what will happen?"
- "What will happen if I let go of this fear? What will this allow me to do that I can't do now?"
- "If this fear were to disappear what would become really important to me?"
- How will life really be different if I lose those last 5kg?

A thought experiment:

Imagine you're alone on a deserted island – you have everything you need to be healthy and well. There are no magazines, no media at all. Nobody is around to judge or critique you and after a while of living off the land and moving your body in fun ways you start to gain weight. There's no risk of anyone ever seeing you. This is your new life and you love it. How would you view this weight gain in this situation?

_____
_____
_____
_____
_____
_____

NAVIGATING FEAR OF WEIGHT GAIN

2. Allow yourself to grieve, feel angry, frustrated etc. This is all part of the journey. Feel the feels and do it anyways. I recommend this article for more on this. https://www.generousplan.com/body-acceptance-grieving-thin-ideal/

3. Show yourself and others some compassion. When you are ready, ask yourself: What might a loving parent say to their child if they were feeling this way? Know that this is a process, keep learning, narrate your life like David Attenborough and remain objective. Be kind to yourself the same way he's kind to all the creatures in the world.

Be mindful of your words around others who may be in bigger bodies How would it make them feel to hear you complain about 'being fat' or 'needing to lose weight". This is only reconfirming the idea that 'fat is bad'. Also, consider this language around your own children. Do you want them to grow up fearing their bodies as well?

4. Diversity your newsfeed. Hopefully, by now you've already done this. If not, today is the day. Ensure your newsfeed shows all different kinds of bodies. Reach out if you need more suggestions.

5. Aim for neutrality: Know that loving yourself 100% isn't instant. It's a journey and we can continue to do the work towards empowered eating on the way. Just being here is a step in the right direction. Begin to focus on what your body can do, the kind of person you are and your values rather than what your body looks like.

6. Connect with your ancestors to redefine beauty. You have come from a long line of strong people who have survived the test of time to bring you here today. What aspects of your own unique beauty come from your ancestors? I have my father's eyes, my great grandmother's skin tone, and my feet turn a bit outwards thanks to my mother's side of the family. All of these things are what make me unique – they are gifts from my ancestors, as is your body. What aspects of your beauty came from your ancestors? If you are adopted and don't know your ancestors, you get to make them up! Remember that we all have ancestors who go back in time to the very first human. If you don't like your ancestors that you know, this is an opportunity to imagine some from the distant past who contributed to all of the things that make you unique.

NAVIGATING FEAR OF WEIGHT GAIN

7. Think of all the things you gain along with the weight:

- ·You are so much happier now that you're not obsessing over every bite of food you put in your mouth.
- You have a lot more time to do things you enjoy because the time suck of dieting is gone.
- You are being more social. You can eat out without fear or worry.
- You are more present with your family and friends rather than distancing yourself or not participating in things that involve food you're afraid to eat.
- You're happier. Seriously. Chronic dieting and disordered eating can do a number on your mental health status and lead to depression, stress, anxiety, and irritability. Sadly, in many cases, it can also lead to eating disorders and suicide.
- You're a bit more fun to be around. Seriously, Not many people like hanging around someone whose #1 priority is to be thin and talks about their diet all day long. It can also be incredibly triggering for some.

8. If you REALLY can't get rid of the fear of weight gain – at least know that dieting isn't a solution. As we've said before. Have all those diets in the past actually helped you achieve long term weight loss? Or was it just temporary? What healthy habits can you focus on instead?

9. Keep learning! Know this is a journey, body acceptance doesn't happen overnight.

10. If you're still struggling, perhaps you've identified that this fear comes from deep-rooted trauma as a child. If that's the case, it may be of value to speak to a HAES aligned therapist or counsellor who can help you to work through this – just as I had to do to work through mine. There is no shame in getting support.

NOTES

_____
_____
_____
_____
_____

MY NOTES

MY NOTES

PRINCIPLE 3
PRESSING PAUSE

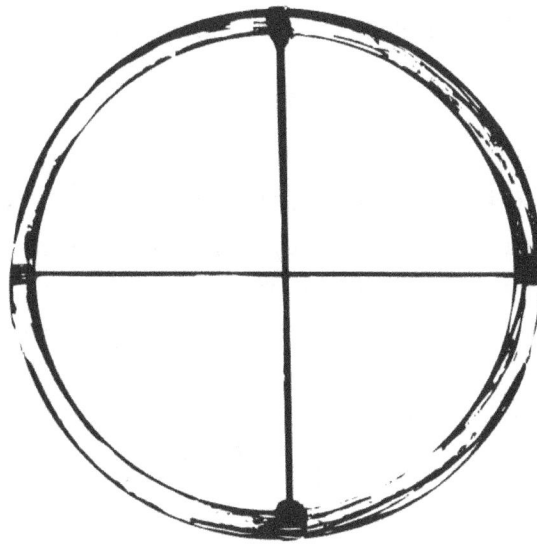

Pressing pause is about stopping before eating to ask yourself if you really are hungry and if not, what it is that you actually need. Empowered Eating will show you how to listen to and honour your body's natural cues so you can eat for not just nourishment but energy and enjoyment as well. This sets the stage for rebuilding trust with food and yourself and making decisions around when and what to eat more of a conscious act.

LISTENING TO YOUR BODY'S MESSAGES

When we overeat, the majority of the time this is coming from an 'unconscious state' or as some call it – A highway hypnosis of food.

We've suddenly realised the food is gone, and we're left wondering how the heck this happened. And it happens, over and over again.

Empowered eating is the opposite. It's learning to press pause so that you can make a conscious decision to eat or not and be in charge of what and how much to eat.

When it comes to overeating this should begin to remove some of the guilt you've experienced because if we consciously make a decision to eat something, there's nothing to feel guilty about! We decided to do it, and that is that. Similar to staying up too late. We may regret it, but we learn from it and we go to bed all the earlier the next day.

If there is one thing that you take away from this course it's awareness. Awareness is a big part of healing your relationship with food, We can also pay attention to what foods make us feel great, which ones satisfy us and which ones aren't as great as we thought. We can also learn what quantity is right for us and say bye-bye to calorie and macro counting for good. Woo!

So how do we do this? I'll be first to admit, this takes a bit of practice but the first step is to pause and ask a very simple question:

Am I Hungry?

If you can press pause and tune in, you're halfway there. I know this isn't always easy though so take it one meal (or bite) at a time. It's about creating a new habit, one that allows you to stop and identify hunger and choose whether or not you want to eat.

We also need to be mindful not to turn this into the "I can only eat when I'm hungry" diet. Being empowered is simply about being able to make conscious choices not attaching any morality to those decisions. After all, that's what got us here in the first place.

AM I HUNGRY?

Recognising hunger is a very basic human skill, something that has been robbed of us through years of diet culture. Some of us might feel we're 'always hungry', while others have long forgotten what hunger feels like.

So, how do you know when you're hungry? What does it feel like for you?

Is it an emptiness in your tummy or grumbling? Perhaps you get headaches and light-headedness? Or maybe, you're like I used to be – when food is needed you get HANGRY! Take a moment to make a list of all the symptoms that you have when you're hungry. What does hunger feel like to you?

Take 5 minutes and write down your own personal symptoms of hunger. If you haven't experienced hunger for a long time, what might you assume it to feel like? What did it feel like in the past?

_____

_____

_____

_____

_____

_____

When you think about all these signs of hunger what do you notice? What do they have in common? These are all physical symptoms – none of them are thought-related or cravings or just wanting to eat for the sake of it. They are genuine signs that your blood sugar is low or your stomach is empty (or both).

AM I HUNGRY?

Simply asking yourself that simple question – "Am I hungry?" and knowing the difference between when you think you want something and when your body is having a physical need is a powerful tool indeed.   If you do pause, and look inward and decide that you are experiencing physical needs to eat, you deserve to do your body a favour and eat something!

When we deny ourselves this physical need we are setting ourselves up for more uncomfortable feelings or worse yet – becoming so hungry that when we get home we raid the cupboard or fridge and eat the entire contents. While morally this is absolutely fine, it can leave us feeling unwell and disempowered.

> *We gasp for air after we have held our breath.*
> *We eat with urgency after we have witheld food.*
>
> *Nina Mills - Feel Good eating*

WHAT IS DOES HUNGER FEEL LIKE?

THE HUNGER AND FULLNESS SCALE.

Once you start to get better at recognising hunger, you'll see that there are different levels. These different levels can help you decide when to start eating and when to stop, depending on how you want to feel. Use this hunger-fullness scale to begin to help identify your hunger levels before, during and after eating. This is simply to bring more awareness into your own body's signals and how different types of foods affect you. Ideally, we would eat at around level 4 - but sometimes life happens!

The Hunger and Fullness Scale

Ravenous	Starving	Hungry	Pangs	Satisfied	Full	Very Full	Discomfort	Stuffed	Sick
1	2	3	4	5	6	7	8	9	10

1. **Ravenous.** Too hungry to care what you eat. During this time there is a high risk of overeating and so if possible we want to avoid getting to this stage.

2. **Starving:** You need food NOW (same as above)

3. **Hungry**: Eating would be pleasurable, but you can wait if you have to.

4. **Hunger pangs**: You're just starting to get a bit hungry and noticing that you're starting to think about food.

5. **Satisfied**: You're content and comfortable. You're not hungry or full.

6. **Full:** You can feel the food in your stomach but it's not uncomfortable as such.

7. **Very full:** Your stomach feels stretched and you feel sleepy and sluggish. You may feel some bloating.

8. **Uncomfortable**: You're 'busting' and you wish you hadn't eaten so much. Some bloating is present.

9. **Stuffed:** Your clothes feel very tight and you're uncomfortable and bloated.

10. **Sick**: You're literally sick or in pain from eating too much.

HONOURING YOUR HUNGER

IF YOUR CAR 'S GAS LIGHT IS ON EMPTY DO YOU KEEP DRIVING?

If you have to go to the toilet - do you second guess that?

No, and no (well at least I hope not) and yet, we tend to do this frequently when food is involved. Over the years we have been robbed of the ability to trust our own bodies.

Rather than eating when we're hungry, which we've already outlined the importance of, eating is often tied to our cognition or based on a set of rules. (Is it lunchtime? Do I deserve to eat? I shouldn't be hungry, I just ate!)

Sometimes when we feel we 'shouldn't be hungry' or we feel we don't deserve to be hungry we will skip meals and ultimately this leads to those feelings of scarcity and restriction that got us into the problem in the first place.

Even non-dieters who go too long without eating will often overeat. All animals do this.

The problem with consistently denying your hunger is twofold. First, it usually leads us to overeat eventually and end up feeling unwell. Secondly, when the mind gets so muted t ignoring hunger signals they begin to fade and you don't hear them anymore. Or you can only 'hear' hunger in extreme ravenous states which can become a self-fulfilling prophecy for all those who feel that they can't be trusted around food.

And so, that's why it's so important if we want to change our relationship with food, that we begin to relearn what hunger feels like and honour that biological need.

Don't be afraid of your hunger. Listen to what it has to tell you. Being hungry means we're alive!

WHEN HUNGER PLAYS TRICKS ON US

Once we get better at identifying hunger we may still sometimes receive mixed messages. Most of the time, even if it's only an hour later, if we think we're hungry we probably are. You wouldn't second guess having to go to the toilet, would you?

What about those times when we 'know' we shouldn't be hungry because we've literally just eaten and yet the overwhelming desire to eat is still nagging? There are some really powerful physical (and not so physical) triggers and situations in general that can skew our body's hunger-fullness signals and being aware of these can help us to make informed decisions around whether or not we'd still like to eat.

1. Thirst:
Our body is clever but has a limited vocabulary at times. Sometimes we have a strong urge to put something in our mouths when really the need is thirst rather than hunger. Imagine you've just had a big lunch before heading to the beach. Shortly after arriving and enjoying some sun, you pass an ice cream vendor. You know you're not hungry but you have an overwhelming urge to consume something – in particular, ice cream. If you can simply pause and ask "Am I Hungry" you may find that you're mouth is dry or other symptoms of thirst are present. Have a drink of water, wait, and ask yourself if you still really want the ice cream. If you do, go for it! But more often than not, it was the thirst that was calling out for moisture. At the very least at least we're hydrating a bit more. And if you still want ice cream - do it!

2. Fatigue:
Did you know that our hunger can increase by up to 25% when we're tired? Sometimes, nothing seems to sustain us, and we're often craving things that will energise us (namely, carbs and coffee). By recognising that this hunger isn't genuine, that your body actually needs rest, you can then be in charge of your next move regardless of what it may be. Just be curious and objective without placing any moral value on it.

3. Hormones:
For women in particular, there is often a time of the month where our cravings and hunger go a bit awol, to say the least. Hunger can increase by up to 17% when leading up to and sometimes during our period. We beat ourselves up for overeating and craving (and consuming) chocolate and other treats. Truth is, our body needs the extra energy it is calling out for and so during those times, the best course is to simply listen and pay attention to our body's needs as making sure that we get enough to eat through the day. If you're hungry eat! Enjoy a variety of nutrients and even some soul food and know that as always, it will all balance itself out the following week.

WHEN HUNGER PLAYS TRICKS ON US

4. Blood sugars:
Sometimes a dip in our blood sugars can produce an overwhelming urge to eat. We feel lightheaded, dizzy, fatigued, and just a little bit 'hangry!' and yet we just ate an hour ago! My own experience with this wasn't enjoyable, I'd panic if I didn't have food at my side 24-7 and was constantly needing to refuel. Sometimes some tweaks to our diet can help manage these highs and lows. This could include being mindful to include fibre and protein with the meals we consume.

5. Stress:
Imagine your body as a survival machine (which it essentially is). If your cortisol is raised and you're in a state of stress whether it's acute or chronic, your body is going to want to accumulate and store energy to protect itself from this unknown danger. Stress is a powerful hunger initiator and recognising what is triggering the stress and coming up with an alternative to soothe other than food when possible is going to help to make some lasting changes and help you feel more in charge of your eating as well as being a positive step for your mental wellbeing.

If you have the urge to eat, go back to the original question in these situations and ask "Am I hungry?" Practice listening to and identifying genuine signs of hunger (gnawing, grumbling, emptiness etc) and check in to see if something else is motivating your desire to eat.

Remember, if you feel like you're hungry - you probably are and so ... eat. The point of Empowered Eating is to learn to trust our bodies again and second-guessing our hunger will only take us farther away from that outcome.

WHAT IF YOU'RE NEVER HUNGRY?

Empowered Eating is all about helping you to reconnect with your feelings of hunger and fullness. As children, we're really good at listening to these feelings. As we get older, these instinctual abilities are robbed from us thanks to many factors.

We're told we need to 'finish our plate' to save all those kids who don't have anything. Or that we should eat it all because we're lucky to have it. Perhaps we have to eat our sandwich before we go play or forgo dessert if our plate isn't spotless.

For adults and even young adults, having a history of yo-yo dieting can seriously mess up our ability to listen to hunger cues which is why it's such an important part of Empowered Eating. By simply asking that powerful question "Am I hungry" we can open ourselves up to so much understanding when it comes to our hunger and the foods that we eat.

But… what if you've asked yourself this question and the answer is always no. What if you just never feel hungry?

There are a couple of reasons for this. It could be that you're not giving yourself enough time to be hungry because you're used to eating by the clock, or you've been told you must have 6 small meals a day for weight loss or maybe you're just eating too much in general.

Perhaps you've taken on a different diet regime and you're increasing your fats and proteins which leaves you feeling fuller for longer.

But what if you're not doing any of the above, what if you're generally not hungry ever?

Unfortunately, repeated dieting and in some cases a disordered relationship with food can leave those feelings of hunger in the dust.

So what should you do if you're never hungry? First of all, if this has become a concern it's always beneficial to speak to a professional who can support you through this. In the meantime, it may be a matter of re-teaching your body what hunger and the act of eating feel like.

Start by setting yourself up with 3 meals a day and a couple of snacks, whether you're hungry or not. I know this goes against the 'eat when you're hungry' idea but drastic times call for drastic measures and we need to ensure that your body is getting the nutrients it needs. By setting yourself up with regular eating patterns again you're simply giving your body a chance to start to recognize these signals again.

Choose the usual nourishing foods when possible; plenty of fruits, veggies, whole grains, protein and healthy fats along with those treat us and nourish our soul. Pay attention and eat even if you just 'think' of eating because that probably means you're hungry.

Sometimes it can be helpful just to be around food and people who are eating. Often we're so busy we don't even think about food which leaves us suddenly starving the next time we see it.

If you're concerned you have a restrictive eating disorder, please speak to your GP or someone you trust. You can also reach out to me at michelle@michelleyandle.com if you need help connecting with someone in your area.

IDENTIFYING UNHELPFUL THOUGHTS

Be mindful of your self-talk – it's a conversation with the universe – David James Lee

The truth is often neglected in our thought processes especially when it comes to the thoughts we have about ourselves and food. Our self-perception has become horribly distorted thanks to thousands of different influences.

We've already identified that our thoughts may need to change. But doing so can be easier said to than done. They are however able to be changed with a little dedication and thought. When it comes to negative thinking there is one question I always ask myself: Is it true? Seems like such a simple question and yet when was the last time you reflected on its answer when it comes to your thinking. Take for example the thought I used to have around sugar.

"If I start, I won't be able to stop"

Is it true? Has there ever been a time when I have stopped after just one piece? Absolutely, it may have been a while ago, but sure, it's happened.

So what's an alternative way of thinking? How can we shift this perception?

"There have been plenty of times where I haven't overeaten or binged on sugar. I've done it before, I can do it again."

Do you see what I did there? It's not about airy-fairy affirmations it's about sorting fact from fiction. I have an analytical brain and when I actually seek truth within my thinking I realise there is so much fiction there I could write a book.

The next time you catch yourself thinking or believing something that is limiting ask yourself that simple question. "Is it true?" And if not, what's an alternative perception you can shift to?

MY NOTES

MY NOTES

PRINCIPLE 4
TUNING IN

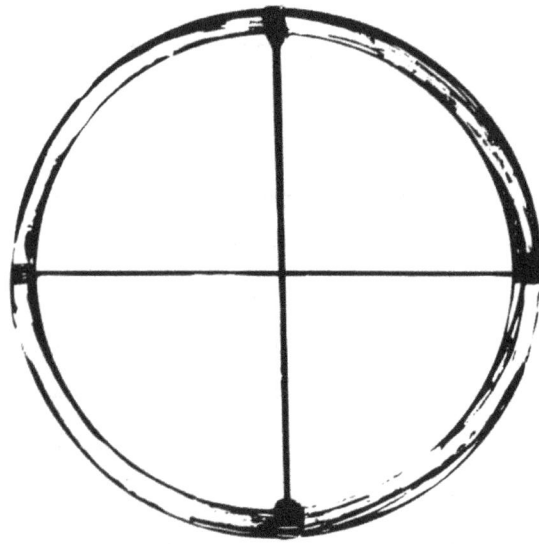

There's power in paying attention to the act of eating. Eating mindfully, slowing down, enjoying our food, feeling fullness and making eating something to enjoy. Tuning in is about giving you the tools to listen to what your body needs as well as increasing the pleasure and satisfaction of eating! Empowered Eating will help you listen to how your body feels after eating and experiment with curiosity rather than rigid rules, so you can feel great before and after eating.

IDENTIFYING FULLNESS

We live in such an extreme world of multi-tasking, high urgency and stress. It gets to a point that even when we're not pressed for time, we're still eating in a distracted state. Maybe we're looking at our phone or the newspaper or using other distractions (driving maybe?)

The issue is that when we eat in a state of distraction, we miss out on the eating experience itself which means that in many cases, eating has to be repeated. It's similar to checking email while you're talking to a friend on the phone. Often, we'll have to go back and re-read the emails because we didn't fully absorb it the first time! Something was missing, just like when we eat in a rushed state and find ourselves needing more. In this case, your friend might tell you you're distracted, but when eating is involved, it's our body telling us so.

I know it's easier said than done but paying attention to your eating while you are in the process of doing so can also help you determine fullness and give you a better idea of what is the right amount of food for you at that time. Slow down, check-in, and keep going if need be.

Everyone is different and so to say that all women a certain age need the same amount of food is simply inaccurate. That's why Empowered Eating techniques that help you to recognise when enough is enough for you, are so important. The hunger scale, your awareness journal and the tips in this workbook will help you with this.

There are a few things you can do to help you determine your levels of satiety. One is to start with the old cliché of using smaller plates*. It can be helpful for some, especially if you're the type to always "clean off your plate" for whatever reason your parents gave you when you were growing up. It doesn't mean that you necessarily need to eat less, it just means that once your smaller plate portion is finished you can stop and reassess before having some more.

Another great strategy and one that we'll dig deeper into is to just slow down while you are eating so that the above techniques actually work. Choose a designated eating location, take some deep breaths, put your fork down between bites or simply become more present with your eating and the food in front of you. This is called Mindful Eating, and we'll be practising this further on in the workbook.

*If using smaller plates is triggering for you - this activity is NOT helpful. Please be mindful of what works for you and what doesn't. Reach out if you need support.

WHAT DOES FULLNESS FEEL LIKE?

REVISITING THE HUNGER / FULLNESS SCALE

The hunger scale can also be used as a guide for determining fullness as well. These different levels help you decide when to start eating but also when to stop, depending on how you want to feel. Again, use this hunger-fullness scale to begin to help identify your fullness levels before, during and after eating. This is simply to bring more awareness into your own body's signals and how different types of foods affect you.

The Hunger and Fullness Scale

Ravenous	Starving	Hungry	Pangs	Satisfied	Full	Very Full	Discomfort	Stuffed	Sick
1	2	3	4	5	6	7	8	9	10

1. **Ravenous.** Too hungry to care what you eat. During this time there is a high risk of overeating and so if possible we want to avoid getting to this stage.

2. **Starving:** You need food NOW (same as above)

3. **Hungry**: Eating would be pleasurable, but you can wait if you have to.

4. **Hunger pangs**: You're just starting to get a bit hungry and noticing that you're starting to think about food.

5. **Satisfied**: You're content and comfortable. You're not hungry or full.

6. **Full:** You can feel the food in your stomach but it's not uncomfortable as such.

7. **Very full:** Your stomach feels stretched and you feel sleepy and sluggish. You may feel some bloating.

8. **Uncomfortable**: You're 'busting' and you wish you hadn't eaten so much. Some bloating is present.

9. **Stuffed:** Your clothes feel very tight and you're uncomfortable and bloated.

10. **Sick**: You're literally sick or in pain from eating too much.

Many of us grew up in an environment that taught us that it was rude not to eat everything on our plates. We may feel guilty and wasteful if we don't finish our dinner, despite being full.

Let this be said: You are NOT obliged to finish eating a food because you took a bite, nor are you obliged to finish your plate despite having had enough. You can always save some for lunch the next day if you'd really like to, or go ahead and compost it.

Also, you have the right to not finish something simply because it doesn't taste as good as you thought it would. Has this ever happened to you? Do you dig into what you think is going to be an epic dessert and find out it's just 'meh'? When we pay attention to our eating we may find this happens more often than not and you are under zero obligation to continue eating it. One of the most empowering aspects of eating intuitively is the ability (and the right) to toss aside food that you don't like. This becomes easier and easier the more you pay attention to the eating process and remind yourself that you can eat this whenever you want to again.

Evelyn Tribole, the author of Intuitive Eating, says:

"If you don't love it, don't eat it, and if you love it, savour it".

In my case, it was saying goodbye to foods like 'low carb bread' (pfft really?) and protein bars that I had convinced myself were delicious. When I really tuned in to what I wanted, these foods lost their appeal and in all honesty, left me wondering what the heck I was thinking!

So, this week I want you really TUNE IN to see how much food you need and whether these foods are satisfying to you. The results might surprise you.

NOTES:

_____
_____
_____
_____
_____
_____
_____
_____
_____
_____

WHAT DO I EAT?

We're going to spend a bit more time on the basics of nutrition in the near future but in the meantime, it's great to have a starting point when it comes to 'what to eat' one that includes a very important principle: The satisfaction factor.

Sadly, over time, we've lost this natural ability to simply know what our body needs and wants. We're constantly bombarded with mixed messages when it comes to food. Bloggers, nutritionists, dieticians, various diets, coaches, all seem to have a different opinion when it comes to what to eat for health so, what are we to do?

The solution is quite simple and it really boils down to 3 questions. The next time you find yourself physically hungry (ie it's not an emotional need). Take a moment to pause and ask yourself these three questions:

1. What do I want?
2. What do I need?
3. What do I have?

Sounds simple right? We've become so used to following external cues when it comes to food that we've lost touch with the basics of how to feed ourselves. And while it is simple, I will be first to admit, it's not always easy. Let's break it down.

1. What do I want?
This question is super important and powerful because if the food we choose isn't satisfying, the need will remain unmet. Have you ever wanted chocolate and decided to have a rice cake instead? Or wanted something salty and grabbed some celery to hold you over? Umm….

When we eat what we actually want, the pleasure that follows will be a powerful force in helping us to feel satisfied and content. When we practice choosing the foods that truly satisfy us, we will find that it takes much less food to decide you've had enough.

So, next time you're making a decision about what to eat, stop and think about all the different possibilities – what is your body craving? Do you want something sweet? Salty? What about texture? Do you want something that is creamy or maybe crunchy? You can also consider temperature. Do you want something cold on a hot day or maybe something hot on a cold one? Do you want something light? Or maybe something more substantial?

2. What do I need?

I believe we all have a basic understanding of what our body needs to be healthy. We know we need a variety of nutrients and fresh whole foods when we can. Asking yourself what you 'need' is an opportunity to think about a variety of outcomes. For example, t's about asking yourself what your body physically needs. For me, I think about how I want to feel afterwards. Do I want to feel energized or am I ok with being a bit sleepy after I eat? Do I want to feel satisfied but not too stuffed? I also think about what I've eaten earlier in the day or the day before because I try to have a variety of foods in my diet. Was yesterday devoid of veggies? Maybe some veggies are in order. Or maybe I've had a lot of grains and carbs and might need some protein.

I also take this time to consider what my health goals are as well as my health history. I have issues with blood sugar so I know that I need to include protein and fibre if I want to remain alert and not cranky. That doesn't' mean I can't have sugar, I just consider this when making my choices. I also think about my goals, so knowing I want to have lots of energy and considering which foods make me feel great. I'm also a busy lady and so I need to be mindful of what foods fill me up for longer so that I'm not always running to the pantry.

3. What do I have?

This is probably the most important because if you don't have it in the house – you can't eat it. It's also why planning is a great form of self-care. The more variety of nutrient-dense foods you have at home the better. That way if you're craving a crisp apple, you have them there.

Stock your home, workplace, car, or purse with all kinds of different foods that can meet all your cravings and nutritional needs. This also comes in handy when you're eating out at a restaurant as sometimes choices can be limited. Consider what you want and need then use that to choose amongst what they have.

Making decisions about food doesn't have to be difficult and some simple planning will definitely help. We all have the innate ability to know what our body needs, and it's sad that diet culture and 'healthism' has led us so astray.

Reclaiming your wisdom isn't always easy but It's there. Be patient and compassionate with yourself and keep checking in.

DIVING DEEPER

Now that we've taken the time to really tune into and enjoy our meals, let's talk about Bio-individuality. This is the idea that each of us is different and that no two bodies are alike. This is why some people thrive on vegetarian diets while others need meat, or why some people feel energised with heaps of carbs and others are left feeling sluggish and tired. We're all different. No one way of eating works for everyone and no food feels and/or tastes amazing for everyone either. Finding out what works for you, in your life, is empowering!

THE BREAKFAST EXPERIMENT

There are various ways to self-experiment and learn what your body loves, this is just about tuning in so we can learn more about what works for us as individuals.
One easy thing you can do is called the breakfast experiment. This is simply choosing 5-7 different types of breakfasts and tuning in to how your body reacts to them. You might choose a higher carb breakfast one day, protein and fat based one another day and then mix things up for the rest.

Here's an example of what a week might look like:

Day 1 Scrambled eggs and a fatty meat such as bacon or avocado,

Day 2 A homemade or store-bought muffin and fruit yoghurt.

Day 3 Porridge with berries

Day 4 Delayed breakfast if you're not hungry

Day 5 Berry smoothie with protein and avocado.

Your week doesn't have to look like this, just try to keep the breakfasts different. Each day, assess how you feel straight after eating and then again in 2 hours time. Do you still feel satisfied? Are you "hangry"? These are all things to consider when figuring out what's best for you. Many people feel more satisfied with a lower carb breakfast, others feel like they need a little more.

THE BREAKFAST EXPERIMENT

Which breakfast/breakfasts worked best for you?

_____

_____

_____

_____

_____

What did you notice about the ones that didn't make you feel great?

_____

_____

_____

_____

_____

My favourite breakfast ideas/recipes

_____

_____

_____

_____

_____

ONE MINDFUL BITE

This is a mindful eating meditation that you can do that takes very little time at all. A big part of 'tuning in' is simply slowing down and paying attention to the food that you're eating so can feel your body's signals but most of all so that you can get the full satisfaction factor.

Mindful eating can be very transformative when it comes to healing our relationship with food. Fiona Sutherland @themindfuldietician first introduced the concept of 1 mindful bite which is really about paying attention to the very first bite of any food that you might eat. This doesn't have to be a specific type of food or meal, it can be absolutely anything.

It's also not about getting it right or being perfect it's simply about engaging with food in a way that honours your body and allows you to get the full pleasure experience.

Mindful eating is a non-judgmental activity.

The first step is to come to your meal or food in a calm manner as many of us are always in a rush. We're busy, or we have kids and so "calm" can be a challenge (and a luxury) I know, but if we can simply go somewhere quiet right before the meal just to take a couple of deep breaths, even if it's in the bathroom, it will be very helpful. Once you've done that, return to wherever you are eating.

As far as location goes, it doesn't really matter either. It's more about settling your body and mind so that you can better experience and digest the food.

Once you've sat down wherever it is and have somehow taken a few deep breaths, you may also consider repeating a mantra or prayer before you dig in. It could be something as simple as 'I am relaxed' or "I am grateful' or "Thank you for this food".

If you're using utensils, consider being mindful about picking the food up. Feel the feels and be aware. If you're using your hands that's cool too – just bring some attention to whatever you use. Now bring your attention to the action of bringing food to your mouth. Just be intuned and connect with that very first taste.

Our first bite can really set up our taste buds. Connecting with that gives us a really good idea of taste, texture, flavour etc.

Following that first bite and as we begin to become more satisfied – the flavours of the food can dull a bit. This can be a signal that you've had enough. Some people find that as the flavour decreases our eating intensifies so tuning in, can help us bring in more awareness.

And so, the idea is that you simply enjoy your first bite and really connect with those flavours. You don't need to do it for the rest of the meal but you absolutely can! Noticing the flavours, or the pleasure of how it feels in your body, whether hunger is dissipating – you can learn so much.

One mindful bite is simply about connecting with the full pleasure of food.

THE FULL EXPERIENCE

There is so much to a bite of food and all of our senses can become engaged. If you want to take things beyond one mindful bite - feel free to dig into the full experience of mindful eating

Sight: Look at your food and imagine you are a Martian scientist. You just arrived on Earth and have never seen this food before. Look at it carefully without naming it. Can you see the water, the rain and the sunlight on the food?

Smell: Bring the food up to your nose. Without naming the scent, experience smelling the food, and then describe what you smell.

Physiological reaction: Now focus on what is going on in your mouth. Begin to notice that saliva is produced, even though you haven't yet put the food in your mouth. Notice the mind/body phenomenon and how the senses respond to the anticipation of food being eaten.

Touch: Now explore how the food feels. Without naming the sensation, just experience touching your food.

Motion and movement: How is it that your hand knows how to move the food directly to the lips? As you bring the food up to your mouth, notice what happens next. The mouth receives the food. Nothing goes into the mouth without it being received. And who or what is doing the receiving? The tongue.

Taste: After becoming aware of the food in your mouth, start biting into it very slowly. Then begin to chew. Notice that the tongue decides which side of the mouth it's going to chew on. Give all your attention to your mouth and take a few bites. Then stop to experience what's happening. What is happening is invariably an explosion of taste. Express what's going on. Be really specific. What is the experience? Is it sweet or sour or juicy? There are hundreds of words to describe the experience of tasting.

Texture: As you continue to chew the tastes change, as does the consistency. At a certain point, you will become aware of the texture of the food because the taste has mostly passed. If the texture causes aversion, you may want to swallow it, but try to keep it in your mouth.

Swallow: Don't swallow it yet. Stay with the impatience and the inborn impulse to swallow. Do not swallow until you detect the impulse to do so. And then observe what is involved in getting the food over to the place where it's going to be swallowed. When you detect the impulse to swallow, follow it down into the stomach, feel your whole body and acknowledge that your body is now exactly one bite heavier.

Breath: Next, pause for a moment or two, and see if you can taste your breath in a similar way. Bring the same quality of attention to the breath that you gave to seeing, feeling, smelling and tasting the food.

Silence: Be silent. By this point, you understand something of what meditation is. It is doing what we do all the time, except we're doing it with attention: directed, moment-to-moment, nonjudgmental attention.

Now, of course, you are not going to do all of this every time you eat! Just enjoy, be aware and notice the experience.

MY NOTES

MY NOTES

PRINCIPLE 5
FALL IN LOVE WITH FOOD

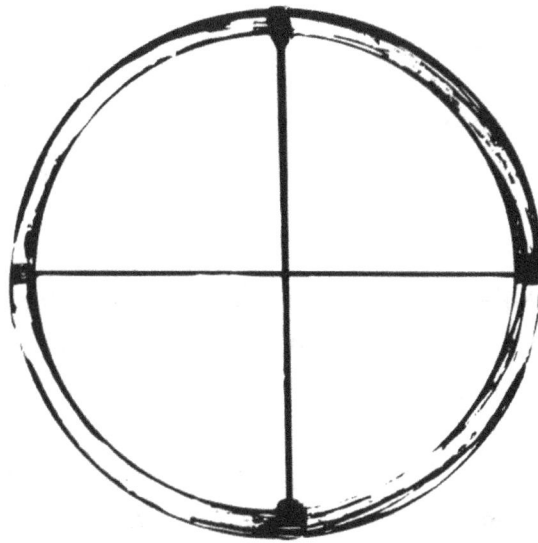

All foods can be part of a healthy way of eating. But the restrictions we often put on our eating can lead to binges and feelings of being out of control. Leaving us feeling guilt, shame and so desperate to count points again. Together, through Empowered Eating, we'll show you how to begin to eat fearlessly again and let go of food rules so that you can feel great AND eat cake (or whatever else you love).

UNCONDITIONAL PERMISSION

Imagine if I were to tell you right now that you could never have _____ (insert favourite food) ever again, starting tomorrow. What would you be doing later today/tonight? I don't know about you but I'm fairly certain I'd be consuming mass amounts of said food.

The same thing happens when we label certain foods as 'bad'. They are given too much power and are naturally the foods that we're going to reach for when we're feeling stressed or rebellious. They provide a release, avoidance and comfort. All foods can be part of a healthy diet and no one food in isolation (unless you have a severe allergy) will cause your health to deteriorate. By labelling certain foods as bad, you're just going to crave them more and overdo it when the stress is too much and you have to have 'just one'.

Enjoy these foods when you 'really and truly want them. Be grateful for the flavours, textures and aromas. Know that you can have these foods whenever you really really really want them. Unconditional permission is a very powerful thing indeed

In case you haven't noticed, completely eliminating foods we think are 'bad' is fairly difficult. They are EVERYWHERE. Our ability to resist them weakens over time and then when we finally get a taste, we feel out of control! Thus labelling foods as 'addictive' and ourselves as weak.

We often have that mindset of 'I already blew it, so I might as well keep going' or we choose to eat it so that it doesn't tempt us later. The more extreme our eating patterns are, the more powerful it will be when we lose our grip. We restrict, we binge and then we do it over and over again.

We've seen this addictive behaviour in animals. When animals are given unlimited exposure to certain foods they enjoy, they don't tend to overeat it. But when we restrict it, watch out!

And so, if we want to change, we need to allow for unconditional permission. If you really want something sweet, have it, enjoy it and be grateful. We've already discussed how these feelings of scarcity can lead to over-consumption.

UNCONDITIONAL PERMISSION

And don't worry, I totally get that this is easier said than done and that it might be scary to have sweet foods in the house again. But I ask you - has restriction or rules ever worked long term?

If you're not ready to have these foods in the house a more ideal transition might be to take yourself out to a café, have an experience, truly enjoy it and know that you can do this whenever you want.

Ultimately, permission takes practice. It's about pausing and checking in and telling yourself:

I can have this, it's an option, really, I'm a grown up!
Do I really want it though?

Think about how it will make you feel, about your hunger levels, about the quality of it and the outcomes.

If you want it – Go for it, seriously! The restriction has gotten you nowhere and we know what will happen eventually. Just eat it, enjoy it. Move on. And yep, this takes practice.

HABITUATION

Chances are if you've ever been on a diet you've got a long list of 'forbidden foods'. These foods will no doubt be the ones you crave, the ones you feel 'addicted' to and ultimately- the ones you lose control with. For as long as these foods remain 'bad' in our minds they will remain exciting and novel to us. The opposite of this is habituation.

Habituation is defined as what happens when you are repeatedly exposed to the same stimulus - whether it's a car, a relationship or food. Eventually, the more we become habituated to this thing, or person - the more the novelty begins to wear off.

Imagine the first time you ever flew on a plane. Everything was so exciting and new! Now imagine you have to fly on a plane daily, or weekly for work purposes. After a while, the novelty wears off. It may still be enjoyable but that level of excitement would have steadily declined.

The same happens with food. Last week I had a delicious meal, and there were so many leftovers! I was excited initially because the meal was so tasty but after the third night in a row, despite still being delicious, let's just way I was looking forward to a change. In a nutshell, the more you eat the same food, the less exciting it is. Sure it still tastes good but it ultimately becomes no big deal.

There have been several studies exploring habituation in relation to food. Even with the most delicious fun foods (Epstein et al. 2009).

The problem with dieting or cutting out particular foods that we're not allergic to is that the habituation effect isn't able to occur. These foods remain forbidden, exciting, enticing and irresistible. Rather than simply enjoying the food, eating it is the start of the eat - repent - repeat cycle that many of us dieters have experienced so many times.

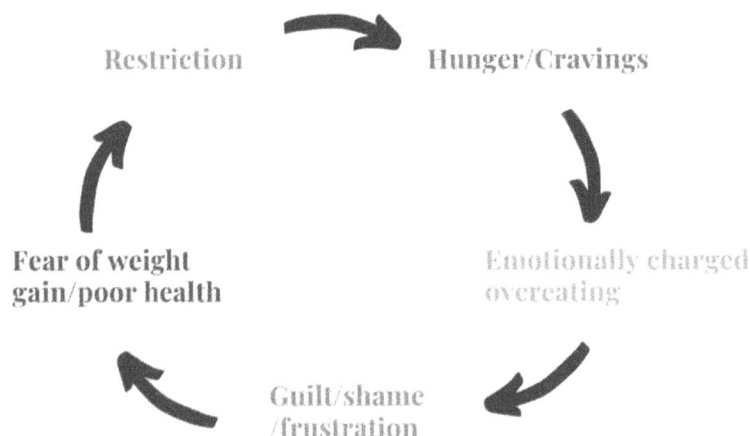

Restriction → Hunger/Cravings → Emotionally charged overeating → Guilt/shame /frustration → Fear of weight gain/poor health → Restriction

SYSTEMATIC HABITUATION

There are many ways to "make peace with food" but it goes much more smoothly if you follow a systematic process using the same food, same brand, and same flavour, before moving on. For example, if you wanted to make peace with ice cream. Choose one flavour, whatever your favourite is, rather than buying a variety of new flavours. Varying the flavour (or even the brand) extends the period of excitement—it's almost like starting anew with each flavour, even though it's the same type of food. The goal of unconditional permission to eat is not to "burn out" on the food so that you'll never eat it again (that is actually a form of deprivation). Rather, the objective is to remove the excitement of the forbidden fruit syndrome.

Prepare to Make the Best of Your Experience

✔ Choose a Specific food (same brand and flavour):

_____

✔ Decide how and where you will eat the food:
____. Home ____ Out ____ Other _____

✔ Decide when you plan to eat it:

_____

✔ What do you need to feel safe? Consider self-care issues and stress:

_____
_____

Check-In:

Before: Take note of how you feel before you (Excitement? Dread? Worry? Curiosity?)

_____
_____

During: How is the taste? Texture? Flavour? Is this taste and flavour meeting your expectations?

_____
_____

After: Any surprises? Overall, did the experience of eating this food meet your expectations? Would you do anything differently?

_____
_____

FEARLESS EATING ACTIVITY

We've already discussed how all foods fit into a healthy diet. Are there foods that you would love to be able to eat without guilt or without binging? If so, here's a fearless eating activity by Dr. Michelle May to help you rebuild trust in your ability to listen to your body's wisdom. Use these steps to help you try one previously forbidden food at a time and eat it regularly until it loses the control it has on you and just go back to enjoying it because it tastes nice. Move through the steps at your own comfort level.

1. Make a list of your "forbidden" or "scary foods, foods that you enjoy but generally restrict yourself from eating.

2. Choose one of the foods from your list and give yourself unconditional permission to eat it when you're hungry and you really really really really want it (the 4 really test).

3. When you're hungry and you decide you want that food, buy, prepare or order one serving.

4. Eat the food mindfully, without distractions and focus on the aroma, appearance, flavour and texture as you eat.

5. Ask yourself, does the food taste as good as you imagined? If you love it, continue to give yourself permission to buy it whenever you (really really really really) want it.

6. Some people choose to have an abundance of that food in their house so you know it will be there if you want it. If this is scary for you, just promise yourself you'll purchase and prepare only as much as you'll need at a restaurant or cafe.

7. Don't be surprised if you want to eat the food all the time at the beginning, that's totally normal. Just relax, the cravings will decrease once you honestly accept that the food is no longer forbidden.

8. When you're ready, choose another food from your list and practice the process again.

9. If you find yourself overeating a certain food again, check in with your thoughts. What were you thinking before eating it? Were you thinking you were naughty, or that you shouldn't eat it? Maybe you were eating it because you thought you'd never get another chance to eat it? These thoughts will continue to drive overeating and bingeing. Try to change these thoughts with alternative perceptions. Fearless thoughts.

10. Repeat. (We'll go into this in more depth later in this section).

THE NOCEBO EFFECT

I assume you've heard of the placebo effect?

Ultimately, it's the idea that if we believe that medication will work – it will, even if that pill is just sugar. Or, perhaps we believe that celery juice will cure half our health conditions and suddenly we feel great. Great Scot! It works!

Today I want to talk about the placebo effect's ugly cousin – The nocebo. In this case, we presume the worse, health-wise, and that's what we get. Now, imagine that a placebo comes with a long list of horrible side effects. The nocebo effect kicks in when we believe that there are unwanted side effects associated with that pill. People have dropped out of studies because the side effects (of the sugar pill) have been so severe. In another example, it was discovered that women who believed that they were prone to heart disease were much more likely to die from it than those with similar risk factors.

The mere suggestion that a drug can cause side effects can become a self-fulfilling prophecy for some. The language used in relation to drug side effects can alter the experience of taking the medication. In a report in the Washington Post in 2002, it was reported that if someone goes into surgery with the willingness to die (perhaps they want to be with their loved one who has passed) they, in nearly 100% of the time, do so. It happens over and over again.

So, I wondered– how is this any different to the believed side effects from eating a certain food? How much of this rise in gluten insensitivity is also related to the increased fear around gluten? It's been shown on several occasions that on a physical level, negative thoughts associated with a particular food can produce a negative physical response.

Let's say that again: IF you believe that a food will make you bloated, tired and unwell, there's a great chance that it will happen, whether you have an intolerance or not.

Meanwhile, we're constantly bombarded with messages from health 'promoters' that gluten is bad, that it will cause this outcome and that, and guess what happens? The perceived threat/outcome is manifested. We hear so much about the power of the mind in relation to placebos and even goal setting and 'manifesting our dreams and so, why is there so little discussion around the power of the mind in relation to how foods can make us feel?

THE NOCEBO EFFECT

The nocebo effect also allows quacks and charlatans to prey on people's worries about food sensitivities. Rather than giving sensible advice to reduce stress, eat more slowly, chew more (all common and simple solutions to gut symptoms), food intolerances are diagnosed, giving the potential for a whole host of income streams: meal plans, supplements, detox protocols and so on." – Plant Based Pixie (Nutritionist)

Imagine you are feeling a bit tired midday. You decide to go get a hair test (which there is no evidence to support by the way) and you're told that you're intolerant to gluten or another food. Suddenly you ditch the food and if eaten again you experience some really shitty side effects. No pun intended. It could be that you are genuinely intolerant but it could also be a matter of 'the power of suggestion'. There have even been cases where people with 'gluten intolerance' have tolerated gluten when they were told there wasn't gluten in it! Isn't the mind phenomenal?

There's still a lot of research to be done but we've seen the effects in studies regarding medication, it would make sense that we have the same outcome with food. I want to be clear, I'm not saying it's all in your head nor am I dismissing genuine food intolerances or celiac disease. Nor am I saying that this is always the case but there is definitely potential that it could happen, just as it has with numerous other similar events.

And so, what do we do about it? For some, some deeper subconscious work may be necessary or maybe some cognitive behavioural therapy techniques. For others, the aim may be to simply be aware of the potential for a nocebo effect, to be objective, to stand back and begin to challenge the charlatans and those beliefs that may not serve you.

So, when tuning into food, also tune into your thoughts around the food. And ask yourself, -can we make space to enjoy this food? To ditch the worry and guilt and actually just appreciate the flavours? The more we practice, the easier it will become. Remain curious and observe the results as you go.

ARE YOU READY?

Right, so hopefully now we understand the benefit of falling in love with food or as Evelyn Tribole, in her book Intuitive Eating refers to "unconditional permission to eat".

It's essentially ending the fight with food and calling a truce knowing that the more we deprive ourselves of certain foods the greater the cravings and often, binging will be. When we give in to the foods we've forbidden the feelings can be so intense that eating will be followed by such intensity that there is no way in hell we can stop at 'just one'.

As we now know, once we've successfully 'overdone it' this leads to feelings of guilt, shame and uncomfortableness followed by the determination to 'start again tomorrow' inevitably continuing the cycle for... eternity.

The effects of scarcity mindset when it comes to food is often called "last supper mentality". Imagine that starting tomorrow you could never have your favourite ice cream ever again. It's been discontinued and will never be re-created. What would you do today? If it were me, I'd go buy as many quantities as I possibly could, stock up and go a bit overboard knowing that this is my 'last chance'. The same thing happens when we deprive ourselves of certain foods that we love. When we restrict them, this creates scarcity and it's our instinct to go 'wild' with a bite following periods of restriction either mentally or physically.
The mere perception that a certain food might become banned can trigger overeating!

This is why it's so important to make peace with food and fall in love with food again.

However, if you're like I once was, the idea sounds lovely but ... how? How do you stop at one biscuit, or, how do you make yourself ok with eating a pack when everyone tells you it's wrong? How can I enjoy previously forbidden foods without that sneaky shame that sneaks up afterwards? We know anxiety-induced restriction isn't good for our health. I just want to eat a f'ing biscuit! I've already shared a couple of activities that can get you started and while everyone has their own answers I can simply share some tips that have worked for me.

Remember, this is something that takes work and time. It's NOT likely going to happen overnight. The longer you've lived in this scarcity mindset around certain foods, the longer it will take. Be compassionate with yourself and take it one day and one food at a time.

Even I don't have it all together. I still catch my old ways of thinking sneaking up on me and have to continually put the work in to retrain our brain. We're trying to clear many many years of conditioning and that shit takes time.

The next few pages are designed to support and guide you to reintroduce formerly forbidden foods back into your diet. If you're wanting to be able to have your favourite foods again without guilt, shame, stress, over analysing, etc and just enjoy it, stick around, do the work and know we are here to support you.

BEFORE YOU BEGIN

Before you get started with any type of food reintroduction, you must ensure that you are

1. Well fed
2. Working with a satisfied tummy.

What this means is, the most important thing to ensure is that when you're reintroducing certain foods using the steps in this book that you have nourished yourself with regular eating that day and not experimenting/reintroducing on an empty stomach. I don't know about you, but when I'm hungry - all reasoning goes out the door. Instead, make sure you've taken the time to eat a variety of foods that day and that your tummy isn't empty. For example, if you're reintroducing chocolate cake - perhaps it's following a good meal so that you feel more in charge of your eating rather than your hungry stomach taking over.

REINTRODUCTION TIPS

1. MAKE A LIST - START WITH THE LESS SCARY STUFF

For some of us, we have a long list of foods that are on our "do not eat' list. Maybe it's gluten-containing foods, maybe it's lollies and sweet treats, maybe you've even banished fruit or sweet veggies. There are so many diets with so many rules it's a wonder we have anything left to eat at all. Take a moment to create a table with three columns. In the first column list all your "a little scary" foods, second column list your "scary" and in the third column your "really scary' foods.

When it comes to reintroducing these foods, start with the less scary ones and go through some of the activities that follow

A LITTLE SCARY	SCARY	REALLY SCARY!
_____	_____	_____
_____	_____	_____
_____	_____	_____
_____	_____	_____
_____	_____	_____
_____	_____	_____
_____	_____	_____

2. GIVE YOUR FOOD THE ATTENTION IT DESERVES

Take a moment to think about foods that you tend to overeat or binge. Can you remember the environment that you usually eat them in? Are you watching TV? Are you on your phone? Are you running around getting lunches packed? More often than not, we're completely distracted when we eat certain foods and this can often lead to disconnection and eating more than we want.

The most important part of reintroducing feared food is to observe. In the next tip, we'll talk a bit more about that but for now, it's important that when we reintroduce these foods into our world that we give them our full attention. Doing so will allow us to thoroughly enjoy the food (seriously, they taste so much better when we pay attention) as well as allow us to observe if there are any negative physical reactions to the food. Surprisingly, when we eat formerly forbidden foods mindfully we might find that we don't enjoy them as much as we thought we did. Suddenly those lollies don't taste as good as you remember… who knew?

So, tip #2 is to practice eating mindfully – pay attention to textures, flavours, colours, and aromas. Most of all. Enjoy it! Yus!

3. EAT WITH GRATITUDE

Whatever you eat, but especially with those feared foods, eat with gratitude. Not in some woo-woo kind of way but genuine, 'wow' gratitude.

When you eat a formerly forbidden food you're likely to still have some negative thoughts pop up full of worry, fear and guilt. I want you to try, just this once, to push them aside and instead while eating mindfully, practice genuine gratitude. If the food tastes good. Enjoy it.

Thank the planet for allowing this incredible food to exist, thank the farmers for their hard work, Say THANK YOU as you enjoy the flavours, textures and aromas. How lucky are we to be able to experience this beautiful food? Practising gratitude and being grateful that I could taste and enjoy amazing food was a huge shift for me.

How lucky are we?!

4. A BEHAVIOURAL EXPERIMENT

By now you'll have created a list of your formerly forbidden foods and you may have already begun to reintroduce these foods intentionally and mindfully as we discussed in tip #2.

Now, I'd like you to go back to your list begin to list the fears that are surrounding those foods. Why did you banish them? Is it because you believe you will gain weight? Become bloated? Be unwell? Maybe you're afraid you won't be able to stop?

Now, once you have listed the foods and why you've avoided them. Start small and observe. Some will start with the whole thing, others will want to start with just a bite.

Remember to eat your food mindfully and give it your full attention. Were you able to stop? How did it taste? Did you even enjoy it as much as you thought you would? Write down some notes in the section at the end of this module.

Remember that if you feel like you did gain weight immediately after eating it's not going to be body fat but potentially water retention. Wait a few days and see how you feel overall. That being said, remember, gaining weight has very little to do with health and is part of what makes bodies unique.

Continue to observe, much like a scientist might observe his subject: Objectively and with curiosity rather than shame or guilt.

5. CHALLENGE DIET/WELLNESS (CULT)URE

We've learned to stop and bring awareness into our eating - now let's stop to take some time to question our beliefs and fears around certain foods.

Does it make sense that one food will make you fat or thin? Heal or harm you? Be toxic or not toxic? Unless you have an allergy – delicious treats do NOT have this much power over you. For the health seekers, if you eat natural foods and home-cooked meals 80% of the time, you're FINE. That one snickers bar is not going to erase all those nutrients. Nor will the dates cause you to be instantly diabetic. In fact, you may find that enjoying treats is actually BETTER for your health holistically.

Challenge these thoughts. Is it true? Is it a fact? Here are some more great questions to ask yourself the next time these thoughts come up:

- Where did this worrying thought come from?

- Who told you it was true?

- Were they a reputable source?

- Do they make money off your belief about this food?

- Has this bad thing associated with the food happened to you personally? (If so, how do you know?)

- Has it happened to someone you know? Do you know this for certain?

- Have you asked multiple medical professionals about your food belief or read other opinions?

- Is this belief that you have about food based in fear? (weight gain, health problems etc.)

- How do you know your fear will become a reality?

- Does this belief you have about food make you happier? Does it increase your quality of life or hurt it?

6. FLEX YOUR GROWNUP MUSCLES

It may seem obvious but, remember, you're a grown-up and can do whatever you want. Amazing isn't it? If anyone comments on what you're eating – eat them too! There really are no laws when it comes to food and food does not have a moral value. You're not a bad person for choosing to have an ice cream or piece of bread – you're a human just like any other that deserves to eat what they want. Just don't steal the ice cream – now that's bad!

7. CONSIDER THE CONTEXT

We tend to view 'treat' foods in isolation - believing we are bad or good based on the self-imposed moral value of that particular food. But as we said before, context is everything. In every case, it's your 'most of the time' that matters. Even too much kale isn't good for our bodies.

Let's say you eat 3 meals a day and maybe one afternoon snack (or more). That is 28 meals. Now, imagine for 2-3 of those meals you end up having something you think is 'bad'.   Look at the big picture when you start to look at the effects of a certain food in isolation. Is one fish and chips meal really blowing 27 other ones? Did you REALLY ruin all that healthy eating or is it your thinking that is the bigger problem?

It's also really beneficial to think about what the food DOES have. For example, bread is not just a 'carb' it has fibre, protein etc. Cheese is not 'fattening' it's protein, calcium and vitamin D and the list goes on...

8. TELL THEM OFF!

It's not an easy task to reintroduce formerly forbidden foods. It can take time and no matter how much we question our thoughts, eat mindfully and gratefully - those thoughts are still going to pop up... a lot.

In Cognitive Behavioural Study there is a method for reducing negative thought patterns called "thought stopping". It's important to stop our thoughts in their tracks because ultimately it's the thoughts that lead to negative feelings followed by the action and then unwanted results. This is referred to as TFAR - Thoughts - Feelings - Actions - Results. So, if we can practice stopping the thought as soon as we are aware of it - we can stop the cycle before it starts.

So, how does "thought stopping" work? As soon as you notice a negative or illogical thought, for example, "I can't eat this, it will make me unhealthy", think or say STOP! It's as simple as that! Once you've stopped the thought - feel free to replace it with something more positive or sensible based on what you've learned in this book.

Just think of all the fun you could have in public places if you shouted "STOP!" out loud?! In all seriousness though, it works for some but it takes practice. Keep challenging those thoughts, give them a good telling-off.

9. AIM FOR SATISFACTION

When you aim to eat foods that truly satisfy you physically and mentally you're able to eat in a way that tastes and feels best in your own unique body. Eating too much doesn't make us feel good, eating too little is also unsatisfying. Eating a chocolate protein bar instead of your favourite delicious chocolate dessert is just going to end up making you continue to crave the thing you actually wanted until you finally indulge (often like a ravenous beast!)

In order to begin to eat for satisfaction, we have to start to practice checking in to see what our body actually wants. This is something that diet culture often takes away from us!

When you're ready to eat your next meal stop, pause and tune in to what you actually want in that time. Do you want something creamy? Crunchy? Spicy? Hot? Cold? Sweet? Bitter? What would hit the spot? Also, consider how you want the food to make you feel. For example, one or two cookies might make you feel great, an entire box might not.

When we aim for satisfaction we are engaging in the ultimate form of self-care.

10. GIVE IT TIME, COMPASSION IS KEY

Please remember that for most of us, we're trying to reverse conditioning that has been a big part of our lives for 10, 20, 30 or more years. I believe the most important tip, THE biggest tip is to be compassionate with yourself and to remember this takes time.

The negative thoughts will keep popping up. Keep challenging them, keep coming back to these tips and keep reminding yourself that this doesn't happen overnight. There is no right or wrong way to begin to reintroduce formerly forbidden foods so you can eat shamelessly.

We also have to start where and we're comfortable. This process could take years and that's ok. For some, it could take weeks. We're all starting at different places and so just keep being kind to yourself and open and engage your questioning mind.

Most importantly, get support. Tell a trusted friend or family member about this process you're undertaking and how it will significantly improve your health and relationship with food. Be open with them, check in with them, and enjoy all the delicious food.

A CHOCOLATE MEDITATION

Here's an activity to take your mindfulness around food to the next level.

Chocolate is a commonly grabbed food in periods of fatigue, stress, sadness and basically, any other emotion that needs comforting.

But chocolate doesn't have to be a 'danger' food. Chocolate can totally be part of a healthy balanced diet and, if you like chocolate, I encourage it! In case it matters, chocolate is full of antioxidants and other health-promoting qualities.

Like a fine wine, chocolate has complexities of flavours, aromas and textures when created properly and like a fine wine, it can be enjoyed fully and gratefully.

Go grab yourself your favourite chocolate or one you've never tried before. It might be dark and flavoursome, organic or fair-trade or, perhaps, cheap and massed produced. If you're not into chocolate, feel free to grab anything off your previous "naughty' list. Are you ready?

---

1. Open the package and take a long deep breath with your eyes closed. Let the aroma fill your senses.

2. Break off a piece and look at it, analyse it, observe it as if you've never seen a piece of chocolate before.

3. Place the chocolate in your mouth and hold it on your tongue letting it melt (if possible). You'll be tempted to suck it but hang on! Did you know chocolate has over 300 different flavours? See how many you can identify.

4. After your chocolate has melted, swallow it slowly and truly experience the textures and tastes as it goes down your throat.

5. Say a silent "thank-you" and truly experience the gratitude that this divine food is on the planet and you're able to experience it.

6. Repeat for as many pieces as you'd like.

How do feel? Is it different from the other times you've eaten chocolate? Did it taste better than usual? Or were you disappointed? Experiment with eating mindfully with other favourite foods.

WORKING THROUGH THE STEPS

1 START WITH A LIST - Make a list of all the foods you've forbidden from least to most scary and begin with those that you feel more comfortable reintroducing.

2. GIVE YOUR FOOD THE ATTENTION IT DESERVES - When eating 'formerly forbidden food' or any food really, try to remove distractions so you can give the experience your full attention.

3. A BEHAVIOURAL EXPERIMENT - List the fears you have around certain foods and begin to experiment objectively. Do your predictions come true?

4. EAT WITH GRATITUDE - Try to push any fear-based thoughts away while eating certain foods and replace them with full gratitude that this yummy food exists.

5. CHALLENGE DIET/WELLNESS 'CULT'URE- Listen to those beliefs you have around food, are they true? Challenge the food police!

6. FLEX YOUR GROWN UP MUSCLES - Remember, you're a grown-up and can do whatever you want! Amazing isn't it? If anyone comments on what you're eating – eat them too!

7. THINK OF THE CONTEXT - Did you really blow an entire day's worth of nourishment by having a few chocolate biscuits? I think not.

8. TELL THEM OFF! When you catch those sneaky negative thoughts popping up - give them a stern telling off. Tell them to STOP and redirect your thinking.

9. AIM FOR SATISFACTION - Stop and listen to what your body actually wants so that you can give in to the full pleasure of eating and satisfaction.

10. GIVE IT TIME - COMPASSION IS KEY - Change takes time, compassion will get you through. This process can take weeks or it can take years -there's no wrong way - you do you.

SATISFACTION IN ACTION

Restriction

↓

Wants a cookie...
but cookies are 'bad' so they have an apple
instead.

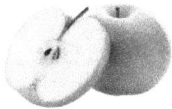

Not satisfied so they have a
'healthier' gluten free low fat
paleo/keto cookie

Still not satisfied. So decides
a couple cookies wont hurt

Eats all the cookies.
Feels guilty

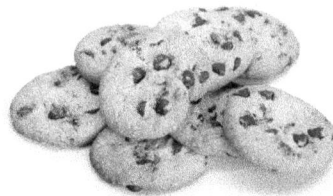

Empowered Eating

↓

Wants a cookie.

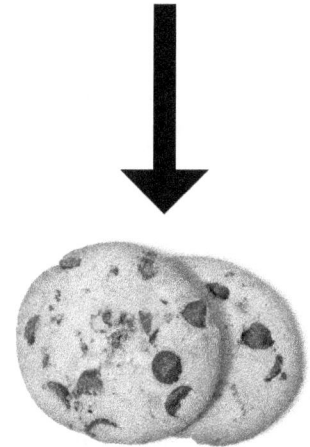

Has a cookie.
or two and moves on

MY NOTES

MY NOTES

PRINCIPLE 6

FEED THE NEED

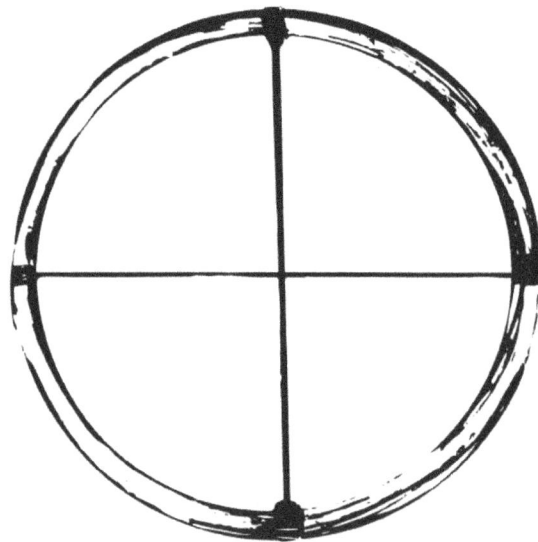

If you're not hungry, to begin with, no amount of food will fill you. Learn new ways to make peace with your emotions. Emotional eating can be a great clue that something's amiss. Together, with Empowered Eating, you'll learn how to tune into what's really going on so that you can start to feed the real need and stop the 'binge-repent-repeat' cycle in its tracks giving you alternative ways to comfort and care for yourself without food.

NOT HUNGRY BUT STILL WANT TO EAT?

So, you've managed to pause and you've asked yourself whether or not you're hungry and the answer came back "no".

But you still want to eat!

These are what we call cravings and I'm sure you know them all too well. They are usually not for broccoli or spinach but something sweet, salty, crunchy or creamy. So what's a girl (or guy) to do?

> *If a craving doesn't come from hunger,*
> *no amount of food will satisfy it*

Ultimately, you have 3 really good options.

The first one is to simply eat. Go for it. Make a conscious decision and enjoy every bite. You ALWAYS have the right to eat. We don't want this to turn into the "I only eat when I'm hungry' diet.

People who eat instinctively and intuitively will sometimes eat when they are not hungry and that's totally ok. I'm not going to turn away a slice of birthday cake just because I'm not hungry. We have to make peace with all eating. Empowered Eating is simply being more aware of our choices so that we can feel more in charge of our eating.

The second option is to distract yourself. It works with kids and often for us adults as well. This is great for those of us who eat when we're bored (but not if you're genuinely hungry) I recommend making a list of "distractions" to help you out when you are craving something and not hungry. Remember though, this should not be housework or something similar because given the choice between housework of chocolate cake… well…

Lastly, try to **figure out what your body is actually craving**. This one is tricky, but with the best results because, if you're not hungry, no amount of food will satisfy you. We'll get into this more soon!

REDIRECTION WORKSHEET

Make a list of redirection activities (see handout). When choosing activities strive to adhere to the following:

- Choose activities that are enjoyable, like a new or favourite hobby.
- Find activities that revitalize, relax or nurture you.
- Choose activities that are "eating incompatible" - so, you can't eat while doing them.
- Make an effort to have some activities that are quick and simple and some that take more time consuming so you'll have all sorts of activities for different situations.
- Be prepared with the things you need to do these activities, have the necessary materials on hand.
- Establish a 'food free zone" at home or at work for these activities.

_____

_____

_____

_____

_____

_____

_____

_____

_____

_____

40 THINGS TO DO BESIDES EAT MINDLESSLY

WRITE IN A JOURNAL

CALL A FRIEND

TALK ABOUT YOUR FEELINGS INTO A RECORDER

CRY

BREATHE DEEPLY

GET A MASSAGE

TALK IT OUT

CONFRONT THE PERSON WHO IS TRIGGERING

DRAW A PICTURE

GARDEN

PLAY WITH YOUR PET

ASK A FRIEND FOR A HUG

WATCH A FUNNY MOVIE

PUNCH A PILLOW

TAKE AN AROMA-THERAPY BATH

GO FOR A RUN

TAKE A YOGA CLASS

SCREAM

TRY A NEW RECIPE

GET OUTDOORS

TAKE A DRIVE

PLAY A GAME ON YOUR SMART PHONE

MEDITATE

SAY A PRAYER

DANCE TO YOUR FAVOURITE SONG

FEEL YOUR FEELINGS

FRESHEN YOUR MAKE-UP

VOLUNTEER

WRITE DOWN 3 THINGS YOU'RE GRATEFUL FOR

WRITE A LETTER

PLAN A DATE TO DO SOMETHING SPECIAL FOR YOURSELF

TAKE A NAP

GET A MANICURE

DO SOMETHING KIND FOR A STRANGER

KNIT

DO A PUZZLE

LISTEN TO YOUR FAVOURITE SONG

ORGANISE YOUR PHOTOS

BUY YOURSELF A PRESENT

DRINK A CUP OF WATER

FEED THE NEED - TRIGGERS!

Awareness is one of the biggest pieces of the puzzle. By simply identifying what's driving your need to feed you can begin to be in charge again. So what's fueling your food thoughts? What's triggering this overwhelming need to eat?

Many professionals refer to them as "triggers". They work much in the same way as any switch would, powering the machine to do what it does. For some, this can have undesirable consequences, especially if you are stuck in an overeating or restrictive eating cycle.

There are several different types of triggers:

Environmental: Environmental triggers happen all the time. They are those amazing morning tea shouts, the birthday parties, the wedding cakes and everything in between. They are stimulated by our senses. Which could also be an advertisement, or simply smelling popcorn at the cinemas.

Behavioural: A behavioural trigger is a repetitive behaviour that causes you to fall into the same potentially problematic eating pattern. These are habits such as always having dessert, or having a 'treat' day whether you want the treat or not.

Physical: Physical triggers are responses to our body's needs. For example, some women find themselves hungrier before their menstrual cycle, or potentially craving certain comfort foods (including chocolate). Another common physical trigger is fatigue. When we're tired, our appetite increases and often we look for those foods which give us a quick pick up.

Cognitive: Cognitive triggers are self-fulfilling prophecies. It's when we have unwanted thought patterns which lead us to overeating and other destructive eating cycles. Thoughts include "I blew it, so I might as well keep going!" or "If I eat one lolly, I can't stop." These beliefs are either true or not depending on the outcome but can be a powerful stimulus for the very destructive behaviour we are trying to avoid.

Emotional: I don't think I need to go into too much detail explaining this one! Stress, loneliness, sadness, and many more emotions often drive our need to feed when we're not actually hungry.

What triggers have you already identified in your own life?

As I've said before, if you're not hungry in the first place, no amount of food will satisfy you. You'll continue to crave, to cave and want that food that is a surrogate for what you truly need.

FEED THE NEED - TRIGGERS!

You've already identified some of your triggers. Now, let's take them one at a time. By coming up with alternatives and practising putting them into action you can begin to feel more intuned to your body and give it what it needs.

We'd probably have to write an encyclopedia series to cover all the different triggers and suitable alternatives but let's look at some of the big ones.

Boredom: I can remember numerous times as a child where I stood in front of the open fridge and got told off by mum. Was I hungry? Nope, bored. So what sort of alternatives are best to beat boredom eating? That's easy, find something to do! Ok maybe not easy, because food will often be easier, but with practice, it's going to be much more fulfilling. Make a list of all the different activities that you enjoy and keep this list handy so you can grab it instead of food in times of boredom. The key is to make them ENJOYABLE activities. If you have the choice between eating chocolate or vacuuming... which will you end up doing?

Rebellion: This is actually a very common one. Many of us eat in rebellion to someone close to them who feels that they should be 'dieting' or at least be cutting back. They sneak in little comments "should you be eating that?" or simply give you that look. So generally, we end up eating in the car, or in another hiding spot as a way of rebelling against that person. This is where boundaries come into play. It's important to talk to your significant other (or parent, sister, etc) and tell them that their comments actually have the opposite effect. In your own time, write a list of what it really is that you want from them. Support? Love? You don't have to give them this list but it will help clarify things for you and get the gears in motion to make it happen.

Stress: I would have to say that 99% of the people who step into my office eat because of stress at one point or another Why? Because they don't call them comfort foods for nothing. Food provides momentary comfort and so when our body needs exactly that, food because the first thing we need when we're stressed.

Loneliness: Many of the people I work with find that evenings are hard for them. They are around people all day and suddenly, you're home alone, or everyone is in bed and so they feel that tinge of sadness that they're alone and decide to comfort themselves with food. This would be a great time to message a friend on Facebook or give them a call. Write that letter to a friend who's been away for a while or grab a good book.

FEED THE NEED - TRIGGERS!

There's also a physical component to this. When we're stressed, our bodies are in flight or flight mode which means it's registering a danger. If our body thinks that we're in danger (perhaps starvation, animal attack who knows?!) it is going to want to store as much energy as it can and increase the need to eat to do so. We're often hungrier when we're stressed and can eat an entire meal and still feel like we need more. So, can I wave a magic wand and make the stress go away? No, but there are plenty of ways to release stress. Deep breathing is at the top of my list what do YOU do to reduce stress?

See-Food: Ah, this is a very powerful environmental trigger. You see food in front of you, in an ad on TV or a billboard, or smell it as you walk down the street. Suddenly – you want it! NOW.

I once had a client who would eat lollies every time she walked by a co-worker's desk because she had them there sitting on her desk. Was she hungry? Not usually. Admittedly she told me she didn't even like those particular lollies but she ate them anyway. The alternative? She asked her co-worker to move the jar somewhere else so that it wasn't in her direct view. She hasn't had one of those lollies since. That's why for some, they may need to remove the foods that you want to avoid from their house until they feel more comfortable. It just simply gives us more time to stop, and check-in. For most of though, it's a much better approach to have an abundance of 'said' food in the house so that we can become habituated. You do you.

FEED THE NEED - TRIGGERS!

Other reasons we might want to eat when we're not actually hungry include:

- We're letting ourselves get too hungry (and then we end up overeating)
- We aren't sure when to stop eating
- We're filling up but not feeling satisfied.
- Just in case I get hungry later?
- The clock says it's breakfast/lunch dinner
- We're not meeting certain needs.
- The food tastes great
- We're worried we might offend someone if we don't eat.
- Our parents always told us to finish everything on our plate
- We eat as a reward.
- We eat because it's there.
- It brings back nice memories.
- We're celebrating
- We ate too fast.

_____

_____

_____

_____

_____

_____

_____

_____

_____

_____

_____

_____

FEED THE NEED WORKSHEET

Ultimately there are hundreds of reasons and it's up to you as an individual to determine what your unique triggers are and come up with an alternative.

Take some time to write down what triggers you've noticed, and brainstorm some possible alternatives.

Trigger: _____

What alternative can I provide that will feed the true need?

_____
_____

Trigger: _____

What alternative can I provide that will feed the true need?

_____
_____

Trigger: _____

What alternative can I provide that will feed the true need?

_____
_____

Trigger: _____

What alternative can I provide that will feed the true need?

_____
_____

Trigger: _____

What alternative can I provide that will feed the true need?

_____

_____

Trigger: _____

What alternative can I provide that will feed the true need?

_____

_____

Trigger: _____

What alternative can I provide that will feed the true need?

_____

_____

Trigger: _____

What alternative can I provide that will feed the true need?

_____

_____

Trigger: _____

What alternative can I provide that will feed the true need?

_____

_____

Trigger: _____

What alternative can I provide that will feed the true need?

_____

_____

DECONSTRUCTING EATING BEHAVIOUR

Some people cope with uncomfortable feelings and unmet needs by eating, binge eating, or food restriction. Many times people are not even aware! These two simple questions pave the way to awareness and ultimately, meaningful change.

What am I feeling, now?

(Refer to this list of feelings, if needed. Or if none if these descriptions seem to fit, try the description, "uncomfortable", and see if that resonates for you).

Fearful	Angry	Sad	Joyful	Disgusted	Surprised	Shame
edgy	exasperated	dejected	amused	appalled	amazed	disgraced
frightend	hostile	gloomy	delighted	contempt	astonished	embarassed
nervous	irritable	grief	gratified	distain	dumbfounded	guilty
scared	outraged	hopeless	happy	indignation	flabbergasted	humiliated
wary	resentful	lonely	satisfied	repulsed	shocked	mortified
worried	vengeful	sorrow	silly	revolted	startled	remorseful

What do I need, right now, to deal with my current feelings?

Refer to ideas below. It's okay if you don't know what you need. The action of being aware, and just checking-in to your possible needs is progress. (If your needs were obvious you wouldn't be turning to food).

Distraction	Support	Deal directly	Self-care
change environment	call a friend	write in your journal	set limites
watch funny movie	email a friend	listen to music	respect vulnerability
Internet	text a friend/	write a letter	have alone time
music	talk to family	sit with your feelings	sleep/rest
go out with a friend	chat online (safely)	reframe your thinking	go for a walk outside
play with your pet	Talk with spiritual advisor	talk to therapist	unplug phone/computer

Original worksheet by Evelyn Tribole www.intuitiveeating.com

COGNITIVE TRIGGERS

So, how can our thinking get in the way of our success when it comes to health?

As I'm sure you've heard before, our thoughts are powerful. It's important to realize that what you believe and think causes you to feel a certain way, which causes you to do certain things, which ultimately leads to specific results. In other words, your thoughts become self-fulfilling prophecies.

Since your results usually reinforce your beliefs and thoughts, this results in the loop we call TFAR: your thoughts lead to your feelings which lead to your actions which lead to your results.

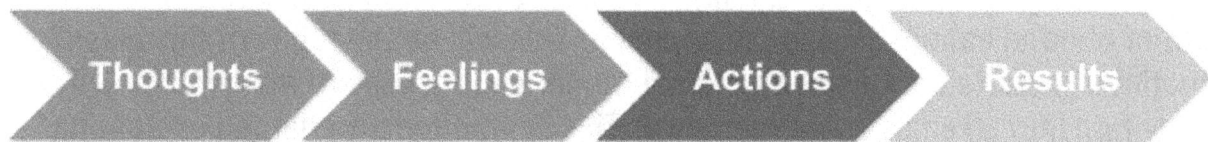

Thoughts > Feelings > Actions > Results

This can be true in all areas of our lives from success to money to food.
It's common for people to try to change the actions and results they don't like without first recognizing and dealing with the beliefs, thoughts, and feelings that led to those unwanted actions and results in the first place.

Thinking thoughts that lead to undesirable results is a habit—a habit that can be changed through awareness. Granted, it's not always easy to recognize when a thought is driving unwanted results, especially if you've been thinking a particular way for a long time. That's where it becomes so important to focus and explore what these thoughts are and where they are coming from.

UNDERSTANDING EMOTIONAL EATING

Before we move on, I wanted to spend a little bit more time on emotional triggers as this is one of the most common concerns for people who overeat. Before I do, it's important to examine the reasons why we eat in the first place. In general, there are three main reasons:

1. <u>Physical hunger.</u> This can range from rumbly tummy to lightheadedness etc. Physical hunger will feel different for different people.

2. <u>Non-emotional: Superfluous eating/overeating</u> – Response to environmental or physical triggers, or food cues, or advertisements, or desserts or popcorn at the movies. There is no emotion attached. You simply want the cake, so you have it. (Most people engage in this at some point or another).

3. <u>Binge eating/ emotional overeating:</u> This is when it becomes a problem: You've heard of Mindful eating? This is the opposite. This will be the focus of this class. Sometimes it starts with a non-emotional trigger but because of many factors, it can quickly turn into an emotional experience. This is emotionally charged overeating. Feeling addicted, out of control, unable to have our favourite treats in the house etc. Firstly, and this is very important to understand. Emotional eating and overeating is not 'bad' and doesn't make you a 'bad' person for doing it! We're simply eating to fill an emotional need. Often it gets a bad rep but it's not wrong in itself, and sometimes even be healthy for example: Eating birthday cake is emotional, communal, spiritual nourishment. Eating to soothe feelings, is normal and ok! As long as you don't feel guilty or find yourself spiralling. We've been eating to soothe since we were babies!

You always have the choice to eat food for comfort, we don't want this to turn into the 'don't eat emotionally diet', because as you'll understand better later - what you resist - persists!

Mindless eating emotionally charged eating, chronic overeating, binge eating – the result is always the same. This is different to emotional eating for the joy of it.

This is the 1 biscuit that turns to 10 or the entire block of chocolate hiding in your car.

Defining it based on quantity is not useful because the amounts are relative to each person. I find it easier to define by cause or motivation: (shame/guilt)

UNDERSTANDING EMOTIONAL EATING

WHY DOES THIS HAPPEN?

There are MANY reasons why this happens but one of the most common triggers for emotionally charged overeating is **a natural reaction to perceived or real deprivation.**

1. <u>Real deprivation:</u> Real deprivation could be due to food scarcity for low-income families etc. Or it could be that we're on a diet and restricting foods that we actually love and enjoy. "I'm not allowed to eat carbs" When you think of overeating, binging, emotional eating in general, we don't often binge to a state of uncomfortableness on things like broccoli, nor do we feel guilty about it. It's almost always something that has been labelled as 'bad'.

2. <u>Emotional /perceived deprivation:</u> You are eating the food but not allowing yourself to enjoy it because it makes you feel guilty. Many people who eat emotionally on occasion do not overeat to the point of severe uncomfortableness followed by intense feelings of guilt or shame. They might have to pop a button here and there but it's not the same as the feelings of 'being out of control' that follow eating something with a restrictive mindset.

As I've said before, restriction (dieting) just doesn't work. So, while the temptation is to put ourselves on another diet to make up for last night's catastrophe, we're simply allowing this restrictive mindset and cycle to continue. Any way of eating that causes you to restrict your favourite foods or label them as 'good or bad' is a diet.

Dieting will only keep you trapped in the cycle and restricting our favourite foods in the name of weight loss will almost always be a driver for overeating. That, combined with emotional triggers, can be a recipe for behaviours we're just not happy with. The first thing we need to do is replace the rules with curiosity, compassion and self-care. That, along with the suggestions in this workbook will help you to feel more in charge of your eating once again.

"Emotionally charged overeating is a natural reaction to perceived or real deprivation."

WORKING THROUGH THE STEPS

On the next page, you'll find a printable page to help guide you through some of the items we've talked about. Go through the process step by step whenever you feel the 'need to feed'.

Let's imagine the following scenario:

You're home, the kids are in bed, your husband is working late. You're feeling the pangs of loneliness starting to creep in and think – I need chocolate.

First, just stop. Maybe you need to put a little note on your cupboard or fridge door to remind you because habits are sometimes hard to break.

Take a breath. Close your eyes – take 5 deep breaths and check in with your body's feelings.

Keep your eyes closed and ask yourself "Am I hungry"?

If the answer is **YES** (the physical symptoms of hunger are there), great! Ask your body what it needs, grab yourself some delicious satisfying food, and sit down at the table (not in front of the television) and enjoy it. Even if your body decides yep, chocolate is what I need.

If the answer is **NO**, definitely not hungry, you have a couple of choices and both are ok. You can decide to eat anyways, repeat the suggestion above. Or, you can simply come up with one of the alternatives you came up with in this chapter .

Remember: Name your emotion and strategize ways to feed the true need. Otherwise, you'll continue to fill the void with food

EMPOWERED EATING ACTION PLAN

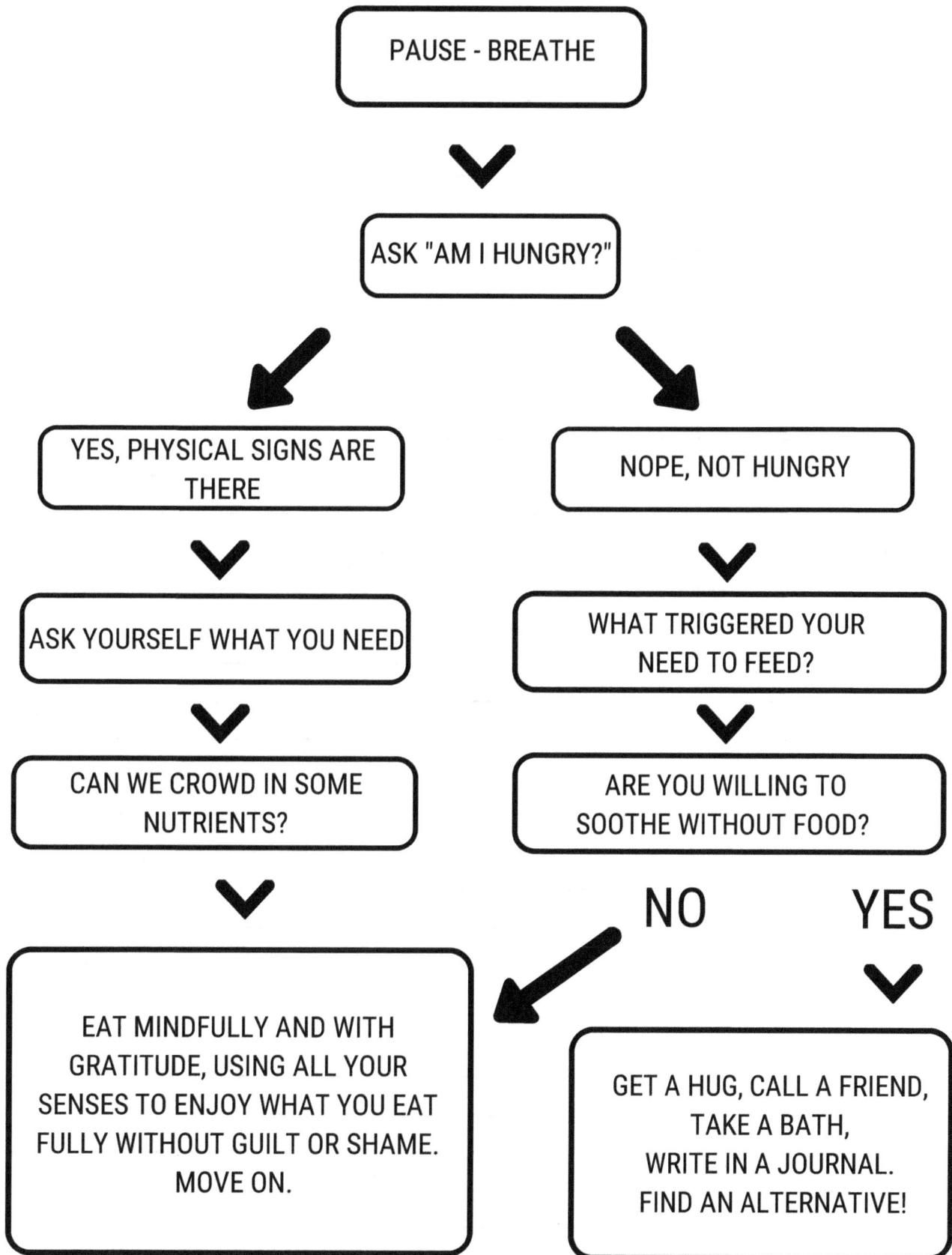

PAUSE - BREATHE

↓

ASK "AM I HUNGRY?"

↙ ↘

YES, PHYSICAL SIGNS ARE THERE

NOPE, NOT HUNGRY

↓

ASK YOURSELF WHAT YOU NEED

WHAT TRIGGERED YOUR NEED TO FEED?

↓

CAN WE CROWD IN SOME NUTRIENTS?

ARE YOU WILLING TO SOOTHE WITHOUT FOOD?

↓

NO   YES

EAT MINDFULLY AND WITH GRATITUDE, USING ALL YOUR SENSES TO ENJOY WHAT YOU EAT FULLY WITHOUT GUILT OR SHAME. MOVE ON.

GET A HUG, CALL A FRIEND, TAKE A BATH, WRITE IN A JOURNAL. FIND AN ALTERNATIVE!

MY NOTES

MY NOTES

PRINCIPLE 7
GENTLE NUTRITION

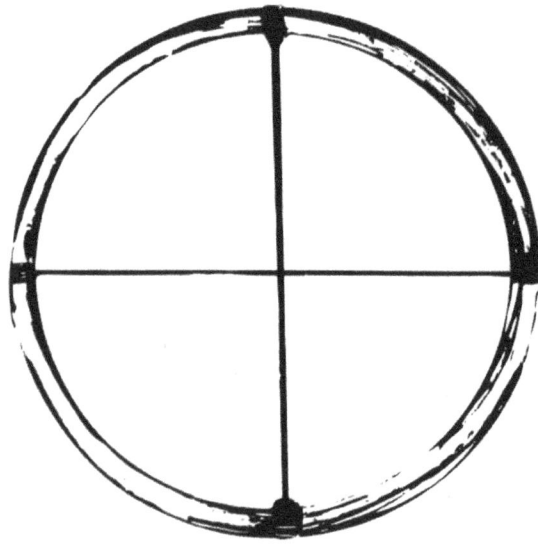

After years of following diets, it's no wonder we're stuck in nutrition confusion. Nourishing our body is important and honouring it is one of many great tools for self-care. But what we choose to eat has got tangled up in what we 'can't' have or 'shouldn't' have. Empowered Eating will help you clear up the nutrition confusion and help you choose more of the foods that make you feel great.

GENTLE NUTRITION

Perhaps you've noticed that there are so many "rules" out there when it comes to nutrition. Everywhere you look, people are telling you to stop eating this or start eating that. They have created so many of these rules that I'm pretty sure there isn't a food on the planet that hasn't been deemed dangerous at some point on the world-wide-web. So what's a person to do?

I believe there should only be one 'rule' and that rule is to start from a place of self-care. Tune out the dieting dogma and turn within. Thank your body for being there for you and ask it what it wants and needs.

Have you ever asked your body what it actually wants? Have you ever asked it if it's hungry before grabbing that biscuit or questioning what it really needs? Our bodies are clever entities – they know what they need for energy, endurance and overall performance. If you take the time to listen to your body's hunger rather than your head you'll find it has a lot of great suggestions.

Essentially, our body needs macronutrients such as fats, proteins, carbs and micronutrients, those little vitamins and minerals that keep everything functioning. Crowd those in as often as possible by simply revolving your meals around fresh or frozen produce, natural proteins and all those healthy fats you're giving your body exactly what it wants and needs and THAT is the ultimate way of thanking our body for what it does for us.

Does it need to be strict? Does it need to be 100% of the time? No way, in fact, eating in a way that allows for those 'soul foods' has been proven over and over again to provide far more lasting health changes as well as a healthier relationship with food.

When it comes to nutrition, think about the foods that make you feel the best physically AND mentally and ultimately, just do your best, whatever that looks like to you each day.

The bottom line is, when it comes to health, what works for one person does not work for everyone and so being able to tune into your own body and make decisions based on that is going to help you to decide what's best for you. Essentially, you can be your own guru!

When it comes to food decisions, try not to think in terms of good or bad, but clearly, some foods make us feel better than others. This is different from person to person. Rather than thinking about what you 'should' and 'shouldn't' do, try asking yourself "What does my body need and want?"

GENTLE NUTRITION

Some questions that you might consider would be: What have I already eaten today? What will I likely eat later? Thinking about these things will help you increase the variety throughout your day.

You will also want to consider your personal health, what specific medical concerns you may have (diabetes, high cholesterol), your family history and any allergies or health goals.

To start, before eating any meal, I encourage you to tune in and ask your body whether it is actually physically hungry (and not just your head saying – eat that.)Once you've done that, whether you're physically hungry or not, follow up by asking your body what it needs. It may be food, it may be comfort or entertainment. If it's food, let's load up on veggies or fruit whenever we can add some protein, whole grains and healthy fats. Do this as often as we can and then relax and enjoy the times in between where you might want something to soothe your soul rather than your physical body.

Gentle nutrition is about focusing on getting more of those foods that our body needs rather than focusing on what we think we 'can't' have. It's about incorporating balance and variety and getting rid of rules when it comes to food.

Begin to be curious about food and try to crowd in some nourishment when you can and increase variety. Maybe even try a new food this week (or two) and let me know how you get on.

CROWDING IN

We all have our own personal (and usually quite long) lists of foods that we avoid because of this reason or that. We're told by both the media and professionals that certain foods are harmful and we need to QUIT them, pronto.

Unfortunately, when we focus on quitting certain foods the same scenario often happens. When we tell someone they can't have something that they love, more often than not, they will begin to crave that food more. This will lead to despair, to eventually giving up and overindulging, which is followed by guilt and shame and the cycle continues. Too often, people are confusing healthy eating with "all or nothing", which ultimately leads to this cycle of restriction/deprivation- surrender then guilt, but it doesn't have to be this way!

What if, we looked at things a bit differently. What if, instead of thinking of which foods you have to give up, we start to focus on what nourishing foods we can add-in?

Crowding-in is a concept I use frequently in my practice. It simply means changing your focus to getting more of the stuff that makes you feel good rather than putting your attention on cutting out the other foods. Focus on increasing natural foods when you can. Even if the rest of your diet doesn't completely change – you're still going to get more nutrients and I believe that eventually, you'll begin to change your taste buds and start to crave foods that your body needs.

What does crowding-in look like? It's is about serving up some new veggies at dinner, adding spinach to your scrambled eggs, or drinking a glass of water before reaching for that sweet snack. Its' about being creative and asking yourself: "How can I crowd in more veggies with this meal?" Or "What might be another oil I could use for cooking"?

This approach, which focuses on taking small daily steps and increasing healthy food rather than avoiding indulgences creates a much more positive framework for implementing lasting change and has been shown over and over again to lead to more lasting results with our health goals. When you add in wholesome nutrient-dense ingredients, your health is going to immediately benefit from the extra vitamins, minerals and antioxidants you're consuming and it can be as simple as adding blueberries to your porridge!

Over the next few pages, I'll be sharing with you tips and tricks for crowding in more colourful veggies, proteins, carbohydrates and fats. While we're at it, why not crowd in a little self-care as well!?

ENJOY YOUR VEGGIES!

So, we've learned all about 'crowding in', or shifting our mindset towards the positive.

If there is one thing that EVERYONE would agree we need to get more of in our diets. It's no doubt vegetables. There are debates over fat, sugar, protein, meat and many others but when it comes to vegetables, everyone seems to get along.

Veggies are nutrition-packed. They have an abundance of micronutrients that just make us feel amazing inside and out. The more variety of vegetables you get each day the better you may feel. By crowding in more veggies, we can enjoy more energy, clearer skin, better concentration and overall feeling fab. Not only that but you're naturally crowding out other options that might make you feel less so.

Government dietary guidelines recommend at least 5 servings of vegetables a day. Ideally, all our plates will be made up with as many veggies as we can get I'd love us all to be having 9+ servings a day but that being said, we are here to do what we can when we can and so there is never any pressure to meet any arbitrary numbers when it comes to getting more veggies. Just enjoy them as often as you can.

So, how do you fit in so many veggies? Do we need to live off salads? Hell no. It's really not as daunting as it sounds and if we grow them ourselves or choose seasonal varieties it doesn't need to cost much either. Here are some common ways I crowed in these tasty gems each day.

Add them to smoothies: Smoothies are the ultimate place to get some veggies. If you really want to go incognito blend into your favourite chocolate smoothie with greens and no one will know. Spinach and silverbeet have a fairly neutral taste so are my top choices when it comes to covert smoothie action. Another trick I enjoy is freezing chopped courgette for smoothies. They make the smoothie creamy and cold without changing the flavour. Making a berry smoothie? Why not add some red capsicum – it adds to the vibrant colour and complements the berries perfectly.

Add to scrambles: Why not give your eggs a boost by adding some greens, mushrooms, tomatoes or capsicums. Sprinkle on some cheese for dramatic effect.

Spiralize: If you haven't got a spiralizer – you totally should! Kids love watching the curly courgette noodles come through the other end (ok I admit it, I love it too) and they make a great addition to your spaghetti bolognese.

Pimp out your rice: Add some chopped greens to your rice in the last 2 min or so of cooking or grate some cauliflower and add to your rice as it cooks.

Add to stews, stews and curries: Finely chop some greens and tell the non-veggie lovers it's fresh herbs – or better yet – add some fresh herbs as well!

Add to your snacks: Simply make a dip with kimchi and coconut yoghurt or hummus and enjoy with carrots, cucumber, capsicum or other dippers. Grab'em while you're chopping dinner.

Squeeze some extra salad onto your burger or sandwich: Burgers and sandwiches are great ways to squash in a few veggies. Load them up with capsicum, lettuce, sprouts, grated carrots... the sky is the limit. Try not to worry about the bun please - it really does taste so much better with one.

ESSENTIAL PROTEIN

We've begun by looking at a variety of ways to crowd in more fibre, vitamins and minerals with veggies and fruit, and today I want to talk to you about protein, why we need it and where to get it.

Whether you're vegan, paleo or neither, protein is essential for our bodies. Protein is found in every cell in your body and plays a role in basic bodily functions from walking to digesting food.

Protein builds, repairs and maintains muscle tissue, can help maintain healthy skin and hair, is involved in the production of enzymes and hormones and can also support your immune system. Protein is referred to as an essential nutrient for a reason!

Protein helps to promote feelings of fullness so that you can feel more satisfied in-between meals. It also has a significant role in keeping your blood sugars balanced throughout your day helping prevent the highs and lows that can occur without.

When it comes to crowding in, how much protein should we be consuming? Ideally, you're eating protein throughout the day at both meals and snacks (if you need them). When it comes to how much, I usually stick to the palm-sized recommendation as a starting point. You may need more, or less, depending on your unique body. You'll find that because of the satiating ability of protein you may not get as hungry as often and your energy is more consistent. Having protein at lunch can also help prevent that dreaded afternoon slump.

Eating a variety of different proteins will improve the likelihood of you getting a complete intake of the amino acids your body needs. This is especially true if you don't eat animal proteins.

If you eat animal protein, I suggest choosing ethically raised meats and fish if that fits within your budget. These may cost more but the importance is the quality of the animal's life and the health of our planet. Of course, this will not be in everyone's budget - just do what you can.

Great vegetarian sources of protein include nuts, seeds (such as chia seeds, sunflower, pumpkin and sesame), legumes, beans, soy and eggs.

There are also some fabulous protein powders available here in New Zealand (and worldwide) that are perfect for smoothies as well as gluten-free baking. My personal favourite is Nuzest New Zealand's Clean Lean Protein, but for those who consume dairy products, whey is another great option.

Play around with different sources, experiment with meat-less days if you'd like, and pay attention to your hunger and energy levels when you make the effort to crowd in some good protein sources.

You are your own guru, listen closely and your body will give you the answers.

FABULOUS FATS

I can vividly remember being a young girl on Weight Watchers happily munching on lollies to my heart's content because they were fat-free. Times have certainly changed, and while I don't believe that sugar needs to be our next scapegoat, it's important that we realise that fat is back, and is super important for our bodies.

Personally, I think a lot of the fat fears stemmed from an increase in processed foods and take-aways. Those types of fats are an entirely different story than the ones that nature produces. People began consuming unimaginable quantities of heavily processed fats in various forms, and like most things, too much of any food can lead to concerns.

Meanwhile, there are some fats that our bodies need and that we should consider crowding-in to our daily routine. These fats are great for our brain, our hair, nails, skin and overall health. They are vital to every single cell in our body as well as being crucial for the absorption of Vitamins A, D, E and K.

There are several different types of fats available to us:

- **Saturated Fat:** Mainly from animal sources such as meat, butter, etc., but also in coconut oil (though it's a medium-chain fatty acid).
- **Trans fats:** While they occur naturally in some foods in small amounts they are more commonly seen in highly processed foods.
- **Monounsaturated fats:** Such as olive oil, sesame oil and safflower oil.
- **Polyunsaturated Fats:** Soy oil, corn oil, and sunflower oil are some examples.
- **Omega 3** are also polyunsaturated fats but are so important I've given them their own category. These include fats from fatty fish and some plants such as flaxseed and chia seeds.

It can all get a bit confusing at times, and so like most things when It comes to nutrition, I like to say – keep it simple.

In general, when it comes to swapping out for more variety I like to stick to cold-pressed oils, natural grass-fed butter, animal fats, nuts seeds and avocados. For those who can tolerate dairy, I suggest full-fat dairy, and cheese rather than the low-fat varieties. Start with all this and you're doing your body a wealth of good. So which fats do I choose most often? I'd say my cupboards are never without olive oil, vegetable oil and butter but for those who want to do a bit more experimenting, here are some more favourites.

Cooking:
For light sautéing, I like to use olive oil, coconut oil, avocado oil, macadamia oil, butter or sesame oil.

For deep frying, I generally use coconut oil or duck fat. If I'm deep-frying doughnuts, however... it will be good ol' canola oil for that.

For drizzling and dressings and smoothies:
Hemp oil, olive oil, flax oil, avocado oil and macadamia oil are great options.

I also recommend everyone take a good quality fish oil supplement if you do not consume fatty fish regularly.

How much fat should we be consuming? It really depends on the person but ultimately, just because fat is important doesn't mean we should have bucket loads of the stuff. A healthy diet is all about balance, variety and moderation, and like most things, with fats, I suggest you get a variety from both plants and animals and pair them up with an abundance of fruits, vegetables and quality proteins.

FILL ME UP FIBRE!

In case you haven't heard, fibre is pretty important. And if there is one thing that most health professionals agree on, it's that we need to make sure we're getting enough.

So what's with fibre? Why is it so important? And how do we get more fibre into our diets?

Let's start by looking at the 'what'. Basically, there are two main types of fibre and that's based on their solubility in water.
It's no surprise then that they are referred to as "soluble and insoluble fibre".
Within that, there are many different kinds as well as some overlapping amongst the two.

So why should we be mindful of the amount of fibre we're consuming?

- If you're trying to keep your digestive system happy and feel more satiated through the day some types of fibre can help. Add in some healthy fats and protein and you've got a winning combo for satiety. Try adding some psyllium or flax seeds to your porridge or simply put a teaspoon or two of chia seeds into your smoothie to reap the benefits if they are in your budget.

Another way that fibre can help support your body and overall health is by feeding the beneficial bacteria in the gut. A healthy digestive system is a happy digestive system. Our gut is essentially the hub of the wheel and by keeping it well populated with beneficial bacteria and feeding the critters regularly we may benefit from more energy, help with blood sugar regulation, immune support and improved brain function.

Ultimately in all these cases, the type of fibre is important and so the bottom line is to strive to get a variety of different sources throughout your day.

My first go-to sources for fibre are fruits and vegetables. Aiming to have 5+ servings a day of veggies plus a couple of servings of fruit is sure to give you a good variety of healthy fibres as well as an abundance of vitamins and minerals.

Some seeds are very rich sources especially chia seeds, which contain 11g fibre per ounce and flax seeds.

Whole grains are a great source of dietary fibre as well. My favourite sources include oats, sourdough bread and buckwheat but there are so many options out there including bulgur, brown rice, quinoa and other grains.

Beans and legumes can also be a great source of fibre. Lentils, chickpeas, beans of all sorts can be added to stews, sauces and salads as a great addition to a balanced diet. I love roasting chickpeas with a bit of salt and paprika. They are SO good straight out of the oven.

If all you did was increase your veggies and enjoy a variety of fruits and whole grains you'd be making great big steps in the right direction when it comes to getting more fibre.

LOVE FROM WITHIN

As part of our gentle nutrition principle, we've been introduced to the 'crowding-in' theory and crowded-in all sorts of different foods necessary to make us happy and healthy. We've crowded in veggies, protein, healthy fats and fibre and today, I want to crowd-in all those amazing microorganisms that populate and feed our gut.

When I say 'the gut' I'm essentially referring to the whole of our digestive system. It starts in the mouth and ends, well, you know where it ends! The gut's main roles are to absorb nutrients and get rid of the things that shouldn't be in our body. If we were a wheel, our gut would be the hub. 80% of our immune system resides there and 90% of serotonin is created within it. Ultimately, if the gut isn't happy, we're not happy!

So what do we need for a healthy gut?

Essentially, three things; a healthy immune system, an intact lining and a good balance of bacteria.

Did you know, that we have more bacteria in our bodies than we do human cells? Overall we've got a couple of kilos of thousands of different strains of bacteria in our bodies at any given time. Diversity is important and the complexity of that diversity is a result of different factors from food to birth to the amount of stress in our lives.

Good bacteria is important for gut health and are like tourists coming and going from our digestive system resort. With that in mind, it's important to continue to repopulate our gut bacteria through the right food and lifestyle choices.

Are supplements necessary? Perhaps in some cases, if we've been through a round of medications or a great deal of stress, but in most cases, I like to start people off with food first. By incorporating probiotic-rich foods as well as prebiotic foods into our everyday diet, we're doing our body (and brain) an abundance of good.

In nutshell – probiotics are the good bacteria that our bodies need and Prebiotics are fibres that your body cannot digest and serve as food for probiotics.

Luckily for us, there is a range of delicious probiotic and prebiotic rich foods that we can crowd into our diet.

Probiotics foods are the fermented goodies including (but not limited to):

- Saurkraut
- Kefir
- Yoghurt
- Kānga pirau
- Kimchi
- Kombucha

Prebiotics are also abundant in the foods we eat!

- Legumes, beans and peas
- Oats
- Bananas
- Berries
- Garlic
- Leeks
- Onions

By managing stress, crowding in fibre-rich veggies as often as possible and adding 1-2 different fermented foods to your diet each day, you're well on your way to keeping your gut great.

Gut health doesn't have to be complicated or extreme in fact, stress in general whether it be related to life or food has just as severe an effect on the overall health of our digestive system.

Keep it simple, show your gut some self care and your gut will love you back.

WHAT ABOUT CARBS!?

Sadly, there's a lot of debate in the nutrition world when it comes to carbohydrates. Everywhere you look carbs are branded as either good or bad and if people have weight loss goals they are often (unnecessarily) told to avoid them. These days it seems carbs are labelled 'bad' more often than good and so what's the deal with carbs? Are they the big bad wolf we're led to believe they are?

Firstly, what are carbs? Are they just potatoes, bread and rice?

Carbs are found in so many foods including dairy products, fruit, vegetables, grains, nuts, legumes, seeds and sugary foods and sweets.

Carbohydrates are made up of three components: fibre, starch, and sugar. Fibre and starch are complex carbs, while sugar is a simple carb. When it comes to carbs, they all have a place in our diets but nutrient-wise, the more complex the carb is, the more nutrients it contains.

Complex carbs have a variety of nutrients depending on the food and more fibre which can fill us up for longer. These include fruit, vegetables, legumes, whole grains and seeds. Almost all centenarians (those who live past 100) have some level of complex carbohydrate-rich foods in their diets. In many cases, more than 60% of their diet comes from carbs. It's certainly not doing them any harm.

To put it simply, (no pun intended) simple carbs are sugars. They burn quickly and can leave you hungry and wanting more. Are they bad? Ultimately, no food is bad or good as we now know. It's what we do most of the time that matters.

How many carbs a person needs depends on a couple of things. Their body's ability to process them and the amount of energy that they burn in a typical day. The more active you are, the more energy you'll burn and complex carbs can definitely be helpful. Carbs are not classified as 'essential' but they can certainly be beneficial... and tasty!

Ultimately, there are some people who metabolise carbs better than others depending on everything from genetics to activity levels and so that's why it's so important to work out what works for you rather than just listen to what has worked for someone else. If too many carbs leave you hungry, tired and grumpy, try having less or swapping out for more complex carbs to see if that makes a difference in your energy or hunger. If not, maybe reducing them will help. Remember though, if you feel restricted this can be unhelpful in the long run. Experiment, try some swapsies and listen to what your body tells you.

All in all, try to avoid looking at carbs as simply 'carbs' try to see all the good stuff they can contain as well. Carbs, like all foods, are not black and white (unless we're talking about rice) and to avoid them completely if they make you feel great, is totally unnecessary.

MICRONUTRIENTS

The foundation of gentle nutrition is understanding that our bodies need certain nutrients to function optimally but is also about being able to balance foods that may not be so nutrient-dense without guilt, shame or anxiety.

We've looked at how to crowd-in essential macronutrients such as protein and fat and beneficial ones such as carbs. We've bulked up on fibre and slow-burning carbs and kept our bellies happy with probiotics. But what about the other little guys, those nutrients that are so small yet so vital to human health?

Micronutrients are the vitamins and minerals that our bodies need to keep us feeling happy and healthy. Unlike macronutrients, you only need a teeny tiny amount to maintain good health.

There are fat-soluble vitamins such ss Vitamins A, D, E and K. and water-soluble vitamins including the B vitamins and vitamin C. There are also minerals such as magnesium, iron, calcium and potassium. All of which are needed to keep you feeling your best.

Deficiencies can have lasting effects on our health in both children and adults and so it's important to pay attention to our bodies and its warning signals when we're not feeling our best.

Governments have recognised the importance of these nutrients and created synthetic supplementation for everything from milk to cereals to orange juice. But are these synthetic vitamins really providing our bodies with the little guys we need?

In most cases, nutrients from whole foods are ideally our first choice. Whether these be plant-based supplements or making sure to get a balanced diet with plenty of colourful vegetables and a variety of protein, fat and carb sources.

Some of my favourite nutrient-dense foods include:

Kale: Jam-packed with an abundance of Vitamin C, Vitamin A, Vitamin K1 and Vitamins B6, Potassium, calcium, magnesium, copper and manganese! Plus there's plenty of fibre as well. Not into kale? Any greens will do. Variety is great.

Garlic: Tastes amazing and is also full of Vitamins C, B1 and B6, Calcium, Potassium, Copper, Manganese and Selenium.

Shell-fish: Clams are one of the best sources of B12 on the planet as well as vitamins C, B-vitamins, Potassium, Selenium and Iron. Oysters also have an abundance of nutrients including zinc.

Potatoes: Surprised? Potatoes actually have a little bit of almost every nutrient we need as well as being incredibly satiating. If you cool potatoes and then reheat or eat cold the next day you've also got a powerful source of resistant starch.

Eggs: I like to refer to eggs as nature's multi-vitamin and most of the vitamins are found in the yolk. They also have healthy fats proteins and are cheap, versatile and taste amazing.

There are so many nutrient-abundant natural foods being grown and raised worldwide but sometimes a good multi-vitamin can be an insurance policy to fill any gaps if your budget allows

When looking for a multi-vitamin there are a few things you should look for when reading the label.

Check that your supplement uses a ready to use folate rather than synthetic folic acid. Many of us can't metabolise synthetic folic acid. It's best to check that it contains natural folate.

I also prefer natural sources of calcium from algae (if vegan/vegetarian) or natural dairy-based sources rather than the lab-produced calcium citrate, carbonate and phosphate used in common multi-vitamins.

When it comes to B-12 (which is essential for brain health and a common deficiency in vegans and vegetarians) you want to look for a form that is already pre-converted and usable by your body. Most supplements use the common cyanocobalamin which is fine if your diet is perfect, stress is non-existent and toxins don't exist. For the rest of us, methylcobalamin is the one you want to look for, it's already converted for you so your body can use it more efficiently.

Same with Vitamin A, beta-carotene can be difficult to for the body to convert in most cases and so look for pre-formed retinyl palmitate instead.

There are some great companies out there that are using these more easily absorbed sources of vitamins and minerals. My personal favourite is Nuzest New Zealand's Good Green Vitality which has all of the above and much more, feel free to use my code MYANDLE to get 20% off, always.

As a general guideline, always try to choose food first if you can but sometimes a quality food-based supplement or something equally as good is a healthy addition to your diet. The most important way to get enough nutrients is to simply eat enough and try to get a variety of different foods. It doesn't have to be expensive or confusing - just do the best you can.

FOOD AND MOOD

By crowding in foods that support your brain, as well as engaging in certain lifestyle changes, you can potentially enhance how you're feeling overall, both mentally and physically. The keyword is potentially as we know there is so much more to consider when we're talking about health.

When it comes to supporting our mental health, try to eat 'natural' food as often as you can. If this was all you did most of the time, you're off to a great start as you're naturally reducing those foods that may leave you feeling poorly. Remember though, eating some processed food that you love and enjoy won't affect your mental health and if you truly enjoy it guilt-free, it can actually help improve it.

When it comes to mood, we can't neglect the role our gut plays. Serotonin the 'happy making' transmitter is formulated in the gut, not the brain, so we will benefit from keeping it happy.

Aiming to get as many 'natural' foods as possible can sometimes be all you need to keep your gut – and yourself happy. Ensuring you include some probiotic foods (kefir, yoghurt, fermented cheeses, sauerkraut, sourdough, kombucha, kimchi etc) into your diet will help to repopulate the mitochondria which can also contribute to a better mood. One study showed that in otherwise healthy people, the right gut bugs enhanced their mood overall and reduced negative thoughts. Julia Rucklidge is somewhere here in New Zealand doing a lot of work in the area of micronutrients and mental health.

Probiotics are just one of many key dietary additions that can help to give our brains what it needs for improved mood. Some other powerful players include the following.

Omega 3s: These are crucial for optimal brain development and function overall. Omega 3s are found in fatty fish and fish oil capsules, nuts, and seeds.

Vitamin D: The sunshine supplement! Have you ever noticed you feel better when the sun is shining? I know I certainly do. The right amount of Vitamin D can positively affect our overall mood. Anyone who has survived a North American winter can attest to that! Vitamin D is required for brain function and development and can be found in fortified cereals, bread, milk and from getting a daily dose of sunshine when possible.

FOOD AND MOOD

Tryptophan: Tryptophan is the key ingredient in making serotonin; without it, serotonin won't be made. Because the body can't make its own tryptophan, we need to try to get it from our diet. There's a reason why it's called an essential amino acid! You'll find it in turkey, eggs, beef, some dairy products and dark leafy vegetables.

So, in conclusion – crowed in a variety of whole foods and you're off to a great start. Experiment with different vegetables, whole grains, proteins and fats and keep note of how you feel*.

Of course, there are so many other influences on our mental health such as lack of connection, stress and fatigue. And while food is not a cure-all, it's a good one to have on the team.

*If you suffer from depression or other mental health-related conditions, please ensure you seek the advice of a dietician, nutritionist or doctor before attempting to treat it with supplements. Always talk to a professional if you are not ok. Most countries have a list of numbers you can call or text for free to get immediate support. Please reach out if you are unable to find your local numbers.

MEAL PLANNING 101

So, you may wonder, if I'm eating intuitively, and ditching diets doesn't that mean I have to ditch the meal prep and planning too?

Absolutely not. It all boils down to intention. When done from the correct space, meal planning is a form of self-care rather than self-control. It's about making your life easier so that you can think less about food and more about getting on with your day and doing what you love.

It's about getting away from rules, calorie counting, rigidity, and making you feel like you've blown it if you go off the plan and embracing meal planning as a way to reduce stress, budget, remembering what to put in your cart and nourishing yourself.

So, how do you meal plan? Well, to be honest, like all things, there is no one way to do a meal plan. I may do mine very differently than what works for you. And sometimes my meal plan doesn't go to plan. Sometimes I leave out 2-3 days on the plan (mostly on weekends) so that it's open to flexibility if we want to go out to eat or have to use up what we've got in the house.

My meal planning actually starts on Monday (the day after shopping day). Because I love looking at recipes online and in books. Throughout the week, whenever I see a recipe I like on social media, I "save" it. There's even a little button on both that allows you to do it. Otherwise, if I see it on the web there are a couple of places that I can store them.

By Saturday, I usually have some new recipes to try along with some favourites. If you already have your own favourites, start there and then you can just keep adding to your favourites list as you go.

I save my favourite meals by writing them down on a word file on my computer. That way I can remember the ones that my husband and I have both loved and go back to them whenever I need them.

Some people just stick to the same thing every week with little flexibility and if that works for you, that's fine too! I love experimenting with new recipes.

I also have to think about when I'm working late. So for example, Monday's used to be a late night for me so I would pick out something simple (sorry honey) that my husband could make or at least get started. On Fridays, as I said before, I usually am just about over it so that's when I get the good ol' reliable ready-roasted chicken and salad meal.

I just draw some columns based on the store or by grouping ingredients and scribble what I plan to eat on the other side. I go through each recipe that I have chosen and read through the ingredients, as soon as I find an ingredient that I don't have, I write it in the appropriate column.

When it comes to breakfast, I usually stick to my favourites and simply keep the ingredients handy. You can write you ideas down for breakfast of course but unless I'm trying something new, I don't tend to. Most days it's either a blueberry smoothie, oats or toast on the weekend. As long as I've got the staples; blueberries, almond milk, eggs, oats, sourdough, peanut butter, protein powder etc. I can make a variety of breakfasts.

Generally, I choose 1-2 snack recipes such as protein balls or muffins to make also but you don't need to. You could just write down some favourite snacks onto your shopping list (nuts, fruit, muesli bars, yoghurt etc) and keep them on hand.

What about lunch? I'm going to be the first to admit that lunch can be tricky. That's why I try hard to make a little bit extra at dinner time so that both my hubby and I have a little bit leftover for lunch. Leftovers are my go-to most days of the week and on other days I'm usually grabbing a sandwich or wrap. Otherwise, good ol' scrambled eggs it is.

This probably sounds really complicated but trust me when I say, I wouldn't do it this way if it was. The entire process probably takes about 30 minutes or less of total planning time on a Saturday night before shopping day. Keep in mind, this is just how I do things - there is no right or wrong way to create a meal plan. You do you!

Meal planning doesn't have to be difficult, time-consuming or rigid. Use it as a baseline, make an effort to have the ingredients on hand and life is just so much easier when it comes to nourishing your body.

The template on the next page is one that I use - I hope it's helpful! Print off or photocopy as many as you need or simply use it as a template to create your own.

SHOPPING LIST

VEGGIES

FRUIT

WHOLE GRAINS

PROTEIN

CONDIMENTS/ OTHER

THIS WEEK'S MEALS AND SNACKS

1:

2:

3:

4:

5:

6:

7:

* Don't forget to plan to make extra so that you're making enough to have some leftovers for lunch each day!

THE BEST DIET FOR ALL?

If you've got a long history of dieting like me, you've probably tried them all. In the 80s, when I started, it was all about Weight Watchers, Richard Simmons and Jenny Craig. Atkins came later then Mediterranean, Slim-Fast, Slimming world, Paleo, detox plans and now Keto is the current craze. We've been told to go low fat, to go low sugar. We've praised the holiness of coconut oil then put it in the realm of the darkest of poisons.

So, what diet is the best?

Which one really works?

If it's weight loss you're after, well, they can all help you achieve that short term. Any calorie-restricted program will. But this comes at a price and usually results in more weight gain which can be discouraging for dieters. So, is it still considered effective if it only works for 6 months? A year? Five years? At what point do we say the diet 'worked'? Plus, we know the negative effects of yo-yo dieting on our metabolism and our health in general.

Often when we inevitably quit the diet. We're taught to blame ourselves, our lack of willpower or self-control. If a diet wored shouldn't you be able to stick to it for life? Wouldn't it actually be the diet's fault if it causes you to 'break' and say 'I just want some freaking carbs!?

So. IS there a diet that works for a lifetime? Sure is. I'm currently on it.

What's the magic formula? In my experience it has to tick the following boxes:

- It's accessible giving your current budget, family's needs, time restraints and lifestyle in general.
- It makes you feel good!
- It's both physically and mentally sustainable.
- It's satisfying and delicious
- It doesn't cause you any type of worry, guilt or stress
- It's flexible, not rigid
- **It's not a diet.**

1. **It's accessible:**

Everyone's lives are different. Some have families of 5, some are single. Some of us have a $250.00 budget for groceries each week, some have $25. Some of us travel often some work from home. Any way of eating that you take on has to fit within your current situation. If your diet is causing you financial stress then it's not sustainable. If it's too hard to find 'said' foods on the road and your job requires you to travel, it's not sustainable. If you are exhausted following a busy day at work and have to spend an extra 45 minutes each night making something that you can fit into your plan while your family sticks to the usual, that may not be sustainable either.

A way of eating that lasts has to be flexible or else, you guessed it — it won't last or won't even be doable, to begin with.

2. **It makes you feel good. Physically AND mentally.**

Most diets, when we start them, do in fact make us feel great. If they don't, as I have said before, they are not sustainable. But we have to remember that health is more than how our body feels. Health is also about how we feel mentally and emotionally. If your diet causes you to feel left out, craving your favourite foods, or any kind of stress at all when it comes to eating out or visiting friends and family then it's not as healthy as we'd like to think and eventually, the cravings become too much and the cycle of 'on again off again' continues.

3. **It's sustainable.**

I know, I keep hammering the 's' word but seriously — for any way of eating to be beneficial, it has to be adherable and to be adherable it needs to be satisfying and delicious, flexible not rigid and never cause you any type of worry, guilt or stress.

The way of eating that you choose has to allow for enjoyment. If you feel deprived in any way, or miss your favourite foods or think "I wish I could eat that" then eventually we will crave and cave. It happens almost every single time. The worst part of this is the shame and guilt that inevitably arrives thus propelling us to begin the cycle all over again.

You may think you're not deprived. Those coconut flour buns might hold you over for now but if you genuinely love a good quality baked bread and have put it in the 'naughty' list, eventually you're going to have some and the feelings that follow that will decide the outcome to follow.

Not only that, but any diet you choose should not only be sustainable mentally but be physically sustainable as well. We can go for quite a long time on a nutrient-deficient diet in some cases but ultimately, eventually, it will catch up with us. As we've learned, our body needs proteins, healthy fats, fibre, and all those delicious little micronutrients. Eventually, a lack in these vital elements that make us healthy, is going to turn that "I feel great" feeling into the opposite at some point. We're humans and there are certain things a human being needs to function optimally. The key is listening to your body and what makes it feel good.

So what's the best diet on the planet? Ultimately, the best diet on the planet is the one that isn't one. It's a way of eating that is accessible, enjoyable and sustainable and provides a variety of nutrients considering your current budget/lifestyle. It's when we're able to listen to our body's signals and eat in a way that makes us feel great.

It's one that enables you to have a piece of cake or freshly baked bread (or whatever else you love to eat) without any guilt, shame or feeling like you need to now 'burn it off' Health is a feeling, not a look.

Healthy eating has to be flexible, enjoyable, compassionate, sustainable, simple and delicious. If it leaves you feeling deprived, even if it's 6 months down the road, then we're simply not going to be able to adhere to it and that's no weakness to you. And, if anyone has a problem with what you eat - feel free to eat them too.

STOP WORRYING ABOUT YOUR HEALTH

I've been 'into health' my entire life. I cannot remember a time when I wasn't completely enthralled with the latest health advice and the latest and best diet. Strolling around a health food store was my idea of a 'good time' and everything I picked up or read excited me – but for the wrong reasons.

I'd like to call it a "healthy obsession" no pun intended. Every choice I made, every book I read, every Facebook post I embraced was coming from the unachievable goal of 'perfect health'. I remember reading somewhere once that food will either harm or heal me. That powerful statement was one I often used myself, and it wasn't until years later I realised that the statement itself often does more harm than good.

You see, the choices I made in the past were not coming from a place of love, they were coming from a place of fear. I was so scared of the glycemic load of oats that I was no longer eating one of my favourite breakfasts. I could only imagine those demonic oats rushing through my body causing insulin to spike and a full-blown war to be fought in my poor body. I'd probably gain a kilo, bloat and all-around feel like crap for the rest of the day. It just wasn't worth the risk. I look at this now and think – for goodness sakes. These are oats – not an episode of Game of Thrones!

Then there was sugar. It wasn't enough to cut out the white stuff, oh no, I had to get rid of the maple syrup, the honey, and the dried fruits. But no, that still wasn't enough. If I wanted to be truly healthy – fruit had to be gone too. Banish the fruit! It will send me into a diabetic coma!! Oh, and we can't forget toxins. Those little nasties are supposedly hiding in everything from fresh farm veggies to toothpaste. Then there were anti-nutrients. I could vividly imagine each little bugger zapping away at my favourite nutrients like full-blown space wars until my body was left depleted and – gasp – unhealthy.

You may think I'm exaggerating – and maybe I am a little, but there is a moral to this story.

The more we worry about health, the more we obsess over it and experience anxiety about it – the further away we are from achieving it.

STOP WORRYING ABOUT YOUR HEALTH

If the thought of going to eat with friends at a less than perfect restaurant causes knots to twist in your gut – that's not healthy. If everyone is eating ice cream on the beach and you're craving it like a madman and thinking about the guilt that will follow, that's not healthy. If you don't eat vegetables because you can't find organic, that's not healthy.

There are no professionals on the planet that will tell you that stress, worry and guilt are healthy and yet it has been socially acceptable to embrace all three when it comes to food.

The hype, the pressures and the conflicting messages are all doing us more harm than good. They are constantly telling us we're not healthy enough. We're not thin enough, we're not smart enough, we're just not enough and they are making heaps of money by doing so. Because of this, we're losing the ability to live life and experience health for what it is. We've lost the intuitive ability to know what is right for our unique bodies, a birthright given to us as human beings. And that, to me, is a tragedy.

You may be wondering 'but if I let go of food rules won't I be letting myself go?' No, you're not letting yourself go - you're letting yourself live!

Those extra 5-10 pounds, that place where your body naturally wants to be - that's your life. That's your late night pizza with your partner, that Sunday morning bottomless brunch, your favourite cupcake in the whole entire world because you wanted to treat yourself. Those 5-10 pounds are your favourite memories, your unforgettable trips, your celebrations of life.

Those extra 5-10 pounds are your spontaneity, your freedom, your love.

- Author unknown

MY NOTES

MY NOTES

PRINCIPLE 8

LIVE THE LIFE YOU CRAVE

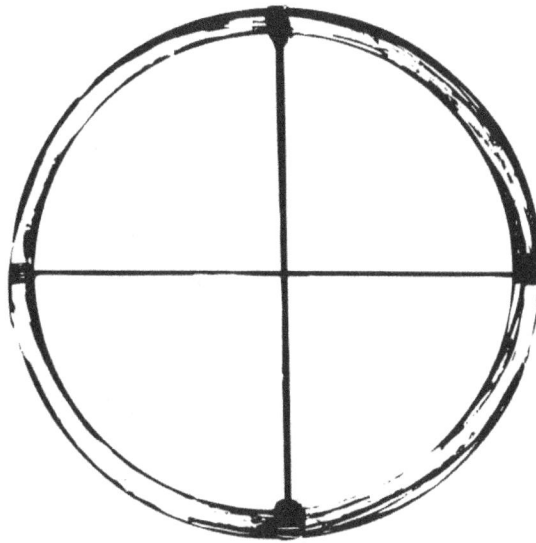

The more we engage in the things that bring us joy and move our body in ways that feel good the less control food will have over us. Empowered Eating shows you a different way to break the diet cycle. Releasing you from obsessive thoughts about food so you can free up the mental space for what really makes you happy. It's time to feel comfortable in your own body, knowing you're respecting, nourishing, and taking care of yourself.

LIVE THE LIFE YOU CRAVE

If you've reached the final principle of the Empowered Eating Workbook congratulations! You may be asking yourself "what now?" That's totally normal! Remember that this is not a diet, so there is nothing to "go off" of. This program is simply about being in charge of your decisions ditching diet dogma and listening to your body.

Following this program (and maybe during) you'll find yourself off track, lured by diet thoughts and shiny meal plans. It reminds me of that ex that you just can't seem to stop texting. Please, don't expect to be perfect, it's not necessary or even possible. We all get off track sometimes, myself included. During those times simply stop and ask yourself again: why? What was it that caused you to get to a point where you felt uncomfortable about your eating in that moment, or that day? Who profits from these emotions?

Use this instance as a non-judgemental learning opportunity. Just like staying up too late, and then going to bed earlier the next day, we can learn from these instances without guilt, shame or fear.

This is a process, not a destination. We're unlearning years of diet culture. We've provided the tools but it's up to you to use them. Some of you might 'get it' right away, for others, it may take more time. All of this is ok. You need to expect that there will be challenges and struggles; perfection doesn't exist. The key is to move forward with self-care and to understand that we are all on different journeys and all unique. Please, whatever you don't turn this into The Empowered Eating Diet. Gasp!
The more you fill your body, heart and spirit up, the less you'll need food to satisfy you. Or, as Dr Michelle May says; Live the life you crave and food will lose its power.

Start by making a list of 10 things that truly make you happy. You might have to go way back to when you were a child. What filled you up? What made you so excited you ignored your mum's calls for dinner? When was the last time you did something on the list? Make it a priority to do at least one of these things as often as possible and watch your need to comfort with food begin to decrease. Remember, you can't pour from an empty cup and if hunger isn't the problem, food will never fix it.

Another activity I highly recommend is purchasing a journal and taking some time to focus each day on what is actually going well and what you love or at least enjoy about your life. Our brains are hard-wired to seek out challenges, mistakes and everything that could go wrong, it's a survival method, but we can learn to focus on the good and retrain our brains. A journal can help with that.

Things that bring me joy:

- ○ _____
- ○ _____
- ○ _____
- ○ _____
- ○ _____
- ○ _____
- ○ _____
- ○ _____
- ○ _____

"Live the life you crave and food will lose its power"

Dr. Michelle May

THE 4 PILLARS: A REVIEW

At the start of this workbook, we learned that health is more than the food we eat or how much we move our bodies. Health is how we feel, but also about the health of our mind, heart, and spirit. It does not mean perfect health but the best health that you can have given your current opportunities and limitations. It's about living our best life. Now, at the end of our workbook, we're coming around 'full circle.

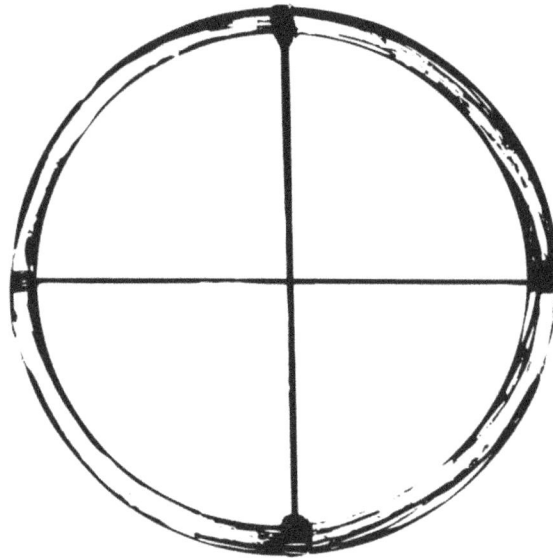

I bring you back now, to The Medicine Wheel.

This symbol is the perfect representation of all the philosophies that I have taken on board and how Empowered Eating involves so much more than what and how we eat.

In review, The Medicine Wheel incorporates the powers of the Four Directions and the interrelatedness of all things. The power of Four Directions is implied whenever a wheel or circle is drawn, since traditional Native American cultures believe everything is interrelated and view life as a continuous cycle that mirrors the changing of the seasons, the daily rising of the sun and the phases of the moon.

THE 4 PILLARS IN ACTION

the east represents the Spiritual, our relationship with nature, our inner-selves, with something higher than ourselves and recognising synchronicity within the universe.

the south represents the Emotional, which includes positive self-image and self-esteem, self-love, self-care and a positive environment.

the west represents the Physical and concerns a balanced diet, movement, sleep, stress management etc.

the north describes the Cognitive or Mental such as learning new hobbies and concepts, connections with friends and family and relationships with the community.

All these must be in balance for wellbeing, and that is also the cornerstone of Empowered Eating.

What can you do to invest in your physical, intellectual, emotional or spiritual wellness?

Brainstorm some behaviours and activities that could contribute to your health and wellness in each area. Remember, this is not a 'to do' list they are simply ideas. It is likely that one or more ideas will jump out at you as a place to start. Take a highlighter and highlight those that do.

PHYSICAL HEALTH AND WELLNESS:

THE 4 PILLARS IN ACTION

MENTAL HEALTH AND WELLNESS:

_____

_____

_____

_____

_____

EMOTIONAL HEALTH AND WELLNESS:

_____

_____

_____

_____

_____

SPIRITUAL HEALTH AND WELLNESS:

_____

_____

_____

_____

VALUES EXERCISE

What are our values? Why are they important? So what's the deal with values? If we are engaging in unwanted habits and behaviours, according to behaviour change expert Dr Mary Grogan, the first step to reprogramming your behaviour is to consciously identify your personal values. A value is a principle, quality or state of being that is important to you. This could be strength, creativity, success or perseverance. Your values form the foundation of who you are (or want to be) and what you do (or want to do).

"Until you make peace with who you are, you will never be content with what you have."
~Doris Mortman

Your core values play a huge part in how you decide to live your life. If you are unhappy with parts of your life—if you are suffering from stress or an illness, and feel generally uneasy in the living of everyday life—then it might be time to go inside yourself and answer honestly two questions "What is important to me?" and "How do I want to live my life?"

Once you start living by your values, life shifts in the most beautiful of ways. You don't hold on to the things that no longer serve you because you have everything you need within yourself.

With your values in place, you can then identify the current habits and parts of your life that don't fit with those values. For example, you might have listed 'freedom' as a value but you're currently in a situation that makes you feel caged in. The following activity will help you to get clear on your values.

1. Determine your core values. From the list on the following page, choose and write down every core value that resonates with you. Do not overthink your selections. As you read through the list, simply write down the words that feel like a core value to you personally. If you think of a value you possess that is not on the list, be sure to write it down as well.

ADAPTED FROM TAPROOT (http://www.taproot.com/archives/37771)

VALUES EXERCISE

Abundance
Acceptance
Accountability
Achievement
Advancement
Adventure
Advocacy
Ambition
Appreciation
Attractiveness
Autonomy
Balance
Being the Best
Benevolence
Boldness
Brilliance
Calmness
Caring
Challenge
Charity
Cheerfulness
Cleverness
Community
Commitment
Compassion
Cooperation
Collaboration
Consistency
Contribution
Creativity
Credibility
Curiosity

Daring
Decisiveness
Dedication
Dependability
Diversity
Empathy
Encouragement
Enthusiasm
Ethics
Excellence
Expressiveness
Fairness
Family
Friendships
Flexibility
Freedom
Fun
Generosity
Grace
Growth
Flexibility
Happiness
Health
Honesty
Humility
Humor
Inclusiveness
Independence
Individuality
Innovation
Inspiration
Intelligence

Intuition
Joy
Kindness
Knowledge
Leadership
Learning
Love
Loyalty
Making a Difference
Mindfulness
Motivation
Optimism
Open-Mindedness
Originality
Passion
Performance
Personal -
Development
Proactive
Professionalism
Quality
Recognition
Risk Taking
Safety
Security
Service
Spirituality
Stability
Peace
Perfection
Playfulness
Popularity
Power

Preparedness
Proactivity
Professionalism
Punctuality
Recognition
Relationships
Reliability
Resilience
Resourcefulness
Responsibility
Responsiveness
Security
Self-Control
Selflessness
Simplicity
Stability
Success
Teamwork
Thankfulness
Thoughtfulness
Traditionalism
Trustworthiness
Understanding
Uniqueness
Usefulness
Versatility
Vision
Warmth
Wealth
Well-Being
Wisdom
Zeal

2. Group all similar values together from the list of values you just created. Group them in a way that makes sense to you, personally. Create a maximum of five groupings. If you have more than five groupings, drop those least important. See the example below.

Abundance	Acceptance	Appreciation	Balance	Cheerfulness
Growth	Compassion	Encouragement	Health	Fun
Wealth	Inclusiveness	Thankfulness	Personal	Happiness
Security	Intuition	Thoughtfulness	Development	Humor
Freedom	Kindness	Mindfulness	Spirituality	Inspiration
Independence	Love		Well-being	Joy
Flexibility	Making a			Optimism
Peace	Difference			Playfulness
	Open-Mindedness			
	Trustworthiness			
	Relationships			

3. Choose one word within each grouping that best represents the label for the entire group. Again, do not overthink your labels. There are no right or wrong answers. You are defining the answer that is right for you. See the example below – the label chosen for the grouping is bolded.

Abundance	Acceptance	Appreciation	Balance	Cheerfulness
Growth	Compassion	Encouragement	Health	Fun
Wealth	Inclusiveness	Thankfulness	Personal	**Happiness**
Security	Intuition	Thoughtfulness	Development	Humor
Freedom	Kindness	**Mindfulness**	Spirituality	Inspiration
Independence	Love		**Well-being**	Joy
Flexibility	**Making a**			Optimism
Peace	**Difference**			Playfulness
	Open-Mindedness			
	Trustworthiness			
	Relationships			

4. My top 5 values are:

COMPASSION

In my opinion, the one thing you need in order to make loving and long-lasting changes to your health behaviours is compassion.

Focus on what you've done right, be compassionate with yourself and you CAN retrain your brain. If you've had a bad day and couldn't be bothered to eat vegetables, it's just one day. The problem arises when we use that one bad day as a reason to continue to self-destruct.

Compassion can move mountains. In a recent study, scientists found that when subjects would show compassion for their perceived failures, they were more likely to keep going and use the circumstance as a learning opportunity.

Another study showed how compassion in dietary choices overall led people to make healthier food choices.

When we talk about self-compassion, one of the founding researchers Margarita Tartakovsky, M.S determined we're talking about three main areas

- Self-kindness: Not being so hard on yourself
- Common humanity: Recognising we're all in this together.
- Mindfulness: Observing and learning without judgement.

It doesn't have to be as complicated as that, though, just think about how you would treat a child if they made a mistake and apply that reasoning to yourself. Just like teaching someone to ride a bike, speak to yourself with encouragement when you 'fall off'. By doing so, you're not only changing the physical stresses that occur under duress, but you're beginning to break free from the dieting cycle once and for all.

More compassion = better health, more kindness and a better world overall.

PRIMARY FOOD

Think back to the last time you were head-over-heels in love. Maybe it's now, maybe years ago. How did you feel when you were in your lover's presence? Me? I felt like I was floating like nothing could go wrong, I was on top of the world! And the last thing on my mind was food, that's for sure.

Children know this feeling all too well. When they are playing and happy, it's a lot harder to get them to come in for dinner, no matter how many times we call them in. When I draw or paint or do other hobbies, I'm so absorbed in what I'm doing that hours can go by without a little hint of a chocolate craving.

Primary foods are what nourish our soul. Whether it's spending time with loved ones, being artistic, walking on the beach or simply reading a good book. When we're completely absorbed in what we're doing and loving what we're doing – physical food becomes secondary. Primary foods go beyond the plate, nurturing us on a deeper level.

Think about the many cultures that use fasting to push secondary foods away while they participate in their spiritual practices. They believe that physical food takes the focus away from the spiritual experience. When we're lacking primary foods we're more likely to turn to secondary ones to make up for the hole its created within. Think about all the times you've been hurting and turned to food for comfort. While there is nothing wrong with eating for comfort (it can be an excellent and easy coping mechanism), we can see that when our lives are out of balance, our eating habits often are too.

On the following page is The Circle of Life. The Circle of Life is a tool that is used in many coaching practices as a way of determining which areas of your life need nurturing. I want you to take some time to consider each area and how satisfied you are with it at this moment. Place a dot on the line depending on your satisfaction levels, closer to the centre means less satisfied and on the peripheries identifies great satisfaction.

Once you've placed a dot on each line, connect the dots and observe your results. What areas of your life need nurturing? What is one action step that you can do this week to increase your satisfaction in one of the areas?

PRIMARY FOOD

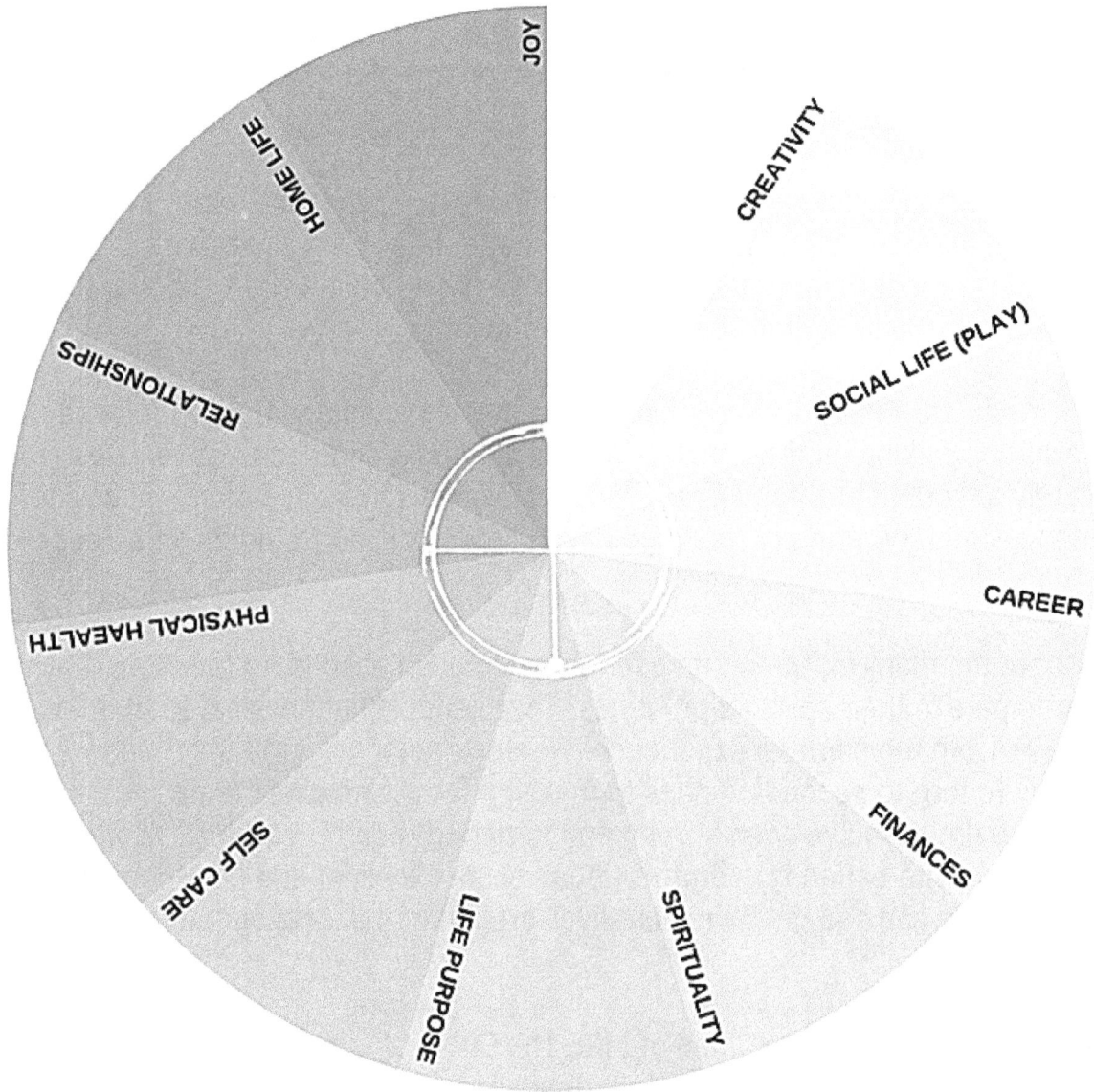

JOY

CREATIVITY

HOME LIFE

SOCIAL LIFE (PLAY)

RELATIONSHIPS

CAREER

PHYSICAL HEALTH

FINANCES

SELF CARE

SPIRITUALITY

LIFE PURPOSE

NOTES:

_____

_____

_____

_____

_____

_____

RECONNECT

In his popular TED talk, Johann Hari famously concludes that the opposite of addiction - whether it be food, drugs, alcohol or any other addictive behaviour is not sobriety - it's connection. There have been countless studies on how disconnect with those around us is often what fuels our feelings of addiction to many things. Feeling connected to someone or something or a group or family is a form of nourishment that we will never get from food.

There are three main ways that we can reconnect; With each other, with our community and with our planet.

Reconnect with each other: Our ancestors may have not had a name for it, but would have valued this source of nourishment. We would have lived together in groups, or tribes if you want to go way back. We would have nourished each other through touch and wouldn't have had the distractions of today's modern world in the form of iPhones and computers. Technology can be a great resource, and very much necessary, but it's not able to replace human contact. I feel sad when I see young people walking through parks with their iPhones in front of them. Or two people who would benefit from talking to each other staring at a screen.

Human touch is one of the most powerful energies in life. Arguably, without it there would be no life! I encourage us to turn off the TVs and computers for at least a short time in the evenings to just talk to our partners, our flatmates and our families. Perhaps you can give your partner a massage or simply hold their hand. If a child isn't touched throughout their lives they won't grow to their full potential. It allows them to feel nourished and valued and adults aren't that much different. We're too busy touching screens and not spending enough time touching each other (not in a creepy way or without consent by the way). We cannot undervalue the importance of human touch. This transference of energy feeds our souls and fills us up. Hugs are a great way to nourish each other. It can be a release of stress or fill us up with the love of a friend. Touch someone's hand while you're talking to them, smile at each other, let each other know they are loved and cared for. I believe this is an important part of what's missing in many people's modern lives. These connections to each other, the community, and the planet.

Reconnect with the community. I remember when I was a little girl walking around my hometown. Whenever I passed someone on the sidewalk I always gave them a "hello" or a smile. I've kept this practice up in my adulthood and I believe this is one of many ways we can connect to each other in our daily lives.

Simply acknowledging someone and smiling at them or saying hello says "I see you" you are worth saying hi to. It makes people feel good, and that bounces right back at you. You may not know that person but you are part of the same community. Be that person who holds the door open for a stranger, or does a kind deed for someone that needs it.

The strength of a community is built upon the strength of the connections between us all. Kindness from strangers - or "random acts of kindness" are the ultimate way to give ourselves and our mental wellbeing a boost.

Another way to reconnect with our community and with food and those who produce it is to visit your local farmers market. There is nothing better, when it comes to shopping for food, than handing money to the person who actually grew your food. It's like saying thank you directly to the person who feeds you. It supports their livelihood and keeps the money within the community. I have met so many people at my local farmers market and crop swaps. I encourage you to seek yours out and find out when and where it happens. Take the time to talk to people, especially those who grow or raise your food. We're getting outside, enjoying fresh air or cool rain and experiencing the elements while we select our food.

Reconnect with the earth. This is a no-brainer really. We all know how much better we feel after a bit of fresh air.

Reconnecting with the earth does not mean that you need to do summersaults in fields of flowers. It's simply about getting outside as much as you can, barefoot when possible and enjoying all of natures wonders. Take the time to listen to the sounds that nature produces, to feel the way the earth feels under your feet and to experience the coolness of the waters.

BODY KINDNESS

I honestly believe the number one way to make peace with food and take care of our bodies is to love and appreciate it. As long as we continue to hate our bodies, taking care of them and eating intuitively is actually really hard. Why would you want to take care of someone or something you hated? You'll also continue to live in fear of foods that might change your body and healing will be increasingly difficult. So how do we begin to be more body positive?

Boosting your body confidence will begin a nurturing experience between yourself and your body and lead to a natural willingness to engage in health-promoting behaviours - as an act of self-care. So, how do we get started?

- Remind yourself you are more than your body. See yourself as a whole human with many talents, qualities, strengths and values. These are what make you YOU, not your clothing size. Focus on what your body can do, rather than what it looks like. People are not going to talk about what a great thigh gap you had at your funeral.

- Ask yourself - what do I love about myself that isn't physical? What value do I bring to the world beyond just my appearance?

- Limit your time on all media, and when on it, ensure that you've diversified your newsfeed as I suggested in principle 2. Diversify your newsfeed with things or people that interest you and connect with your core values. Remember, you're in control of what appears on your social media feed.

- Create strong and affirming positive statements: These can be powerful weapons to combat unhelpful body comparisons. Some you might like to try include, "I am enough", "I am more than my body", "I deserve to nourish and take care of myself". Think about what resonates for you and keep this somewhere where you will see it often.

- Nurture your whole self: Practice body kindness, mindfulness, and self-care. Eat, and move in ways that make you feel GOOD.

- Be realistic: No one feels great about their body all of the time. Poor body image moments happen; it's important we don't respond to negative feelings with unhelpful behaviours.

I highly recommend the book: **The Body is Not an Apology** by Sonya Renee Taylor as well as **The Body is Not an Apology Workbook**. Sonya's thought-provoking book and workbook will give you clear action steps to begin the journey of radical self-love and making the world a better place for all of us.

Another great book is: **Embody: Learning to Love Your Unique Body (and Quiet that Critical Voice!)** by Connie Sobczak. I've also added some of my other favourites to the back of this workbook.

MOVING YOUR BODY

If there's one thing everyone can agree with - it's the importance of moving our bodies. Not only can it be beneficial for many health issues but it can also increase our energy levels, concentration and reduce stress. Sounds great right? So why are less and less people doing it consistently?

There are many barriers to exercise and each of them is individual however a common one that I encounter is that exercise has been seen solely as a way to balance calorie intake and expenditure. Boring! We do movement as a way to become, or stay slim and ultimately as punishment for being in a bigger body. Because of this, we may choose exercises that don't bring us enjoyment they are simply a means to a neverending end. Now that does not sound like a lot of fun to me.

There are of course many other barriers to daily movement many of which include lack of time. It's not an excuse so don't beat yourself up over it - it's just a simple fact. We are busier and busier in these modern times and things show no sign of slowing down. In that case, it can be great to try to fit movement into our day as opposed to trying to fit in a time that does not exist. If all you did was one thing I'd start with just being mindful to sit less and move more. Whatever that looks like for you. For example, most of my day is spent sitting down so I set an alarm to go off every hour so I can get up, stretch, squat, check the mailbox, play with the cats or anything else to get the blood circulating.

It's also important to distinguish between exercise (which honestly reminds me of the 80s aerobics classes I used to partake in) and movement. The World Health Organization in fact emphasizes that physical activity does not mean only exercise or sports (2010) but can include a whole host of other activities such as playing, gardening, doing chores, dancing and recreational activities.

Bottom line, if we're going to begin increasing exercise, it has to be pleasurable not punishment. No pain - no gain is so 1990s.

How does moving your body make you feel? Pleasurable movement should:

- be rejuvenating rather than exhausting us.
- enhance the connection to mind and body.
- Alleviates stress rather than amplifying it.
- Provides genuine enjoyment and pleasure.

What sort of activities do you enjoy doing? What did you love to do as a child? How long has it been since you actually enjoyed exercise? The worksheet on the following page will help you to get clear on what you enjoy and what you don't and hopefully give you some new ideas as well.

Ultimately, when it comes to movement - do what you can, make it enjoyable or functional and do it consistently.

MOVING YOUR BODY

Activity	Interest 1/10	Activity	Interest 1/10	Activity	Interest 1/10
Badminton		YouTube workouts		Laser tag	
Basketball		Ripper Rugby		Kayaking	
Cycling		Gardening		Dragon boating	
Paddleboarding		Geocoaching		Martial Arts	
Surfing		Gymnastics		Paintball	
Bodyboarding		Hiking		Pilates	
Skiing		Hulahooping		Ping pong	
Dancing		Ice or roller skating		Playing with pets	
Zumba		Jumping rope		Playing with kids	
Yoga		Weight lifting		Football	
Rock climbing		Tennis			
Running		Trampoline			
Sailing		Dance or fitness video games			
Skateboarding		Volleyball			
Snowboarding		Wakeboarding			
Golfing		Walking			
Soccor		Cross fit			
Swimming		Running			
Rugby		Netball			

SELF CARE ASSESSMENT

I've said it once and I'll say it again - and again and again. Self-care is so important. If we have an unhealthy relationship with food - self-care is going to be a big part of healing it. Self-care is not all about spa days and manicures and it looks different to everyone. It could be anything from setting boundaries to brushing your teeth.

This assessment will help you to think about how frequently and how well you are engaging in various self-care activities. It will also help you to look for patterns and help you to identify any gaps.

This list is just a starting point to get you thinking about your own self-care needs and there's no wrong way to do this. I understand that some of these activities may not be of interest to you. It's all about reconnecting with what does appeal.

As you go through the various self-care activities - tick the box under the number or star that would correspond to where you are at at the moment and then go back and tick the box under the medicine wheel if it's something you'd like to work on.

1	I do this poorly/ I rarely do this
2	I do this ok/ I do it sometimes
3	I do this well/ I do it often
⊕	I would like to improve this

**Based on a similar assessment from Therapist Aid.

SELF CARE ASSESSMENT

1 2 3 ⊕ **Physical self care**

- ☐☐☐ ☐ Eating nourishing foods
- ☐☐☐ ☐ Looking after my personal hygene
- ☐☐☐ ☐ Engaging in physical activity
- ☐☐☐ ☐ Wearing clothes that make me feel good about myself
- ☐☐☐ ☐ Engaging in physical activity that I LOVE
- ☐☐☐ ☐ Eating regular meals - honouring hunger
- ☐☐☐ ☐ Getting enough sleep
- ☐☐☐ ☐ Regular preventative medical appointments (teeth clean, check ups)
- ☐☐☐ ☐ Taking a 'sick day' when sick and getting rest
- ☐☐☐ ☐ Drinking water regularly through my day
- ☐☐☐ ☐ **Overall physical self care**

1 2 3 ⊕ **Psychological/ Emotional self care**

- ☐☐☐ ☐ Taking time off from work/school or other obligations
- ☐☐☐ ☐ Participating in hobbies I enjoy
- ☐☐☐ ☐ Getting away from distractions (phone, tablet, email etc.)
- ☐☐☐ ☐ Learning new things, outside of work or school
- ☐☐☐ ☐ Expressing my feelings in healthy ways (journalling, art, talking etc.)
- ☐☐☐ ☐ Recognising my own strenghts and achievements
- ☐☐☐ ☐ Making time for vacations or day trips
- ☐☐☐ ☐ Doing activities that are comforting (taking a bath, reading etc.)
- ☐☐☐ ☐ Finding reasons to laugh
- ☐☐☐ ☐ Talking about my problems with someone who cares
- ☐☐☐ ☐ **Overall psychological/emotional wellbeing**

SELF CARE ASSESSMENT

1 2 3 ⊕ Social self care

- ☐☐☐ ☐ Spending time with people I like
- ☐☐☐ ☐ Calling or writing to friends and family who are far away
- ☐☐☐ ☐ Engaging in stimulating conversations
- ☐☐☐ ☐ Meeting new people
- ☐☐☐ ☐ Spending time alone with my romantic partner
- ☐☐☐ ☐ Asking others for help when needed
- ☐☐☐ ☐ Doing enjoyable activities with other people
- ☐☐☐ ☐ Making time for intimate activities with my partner
- ☐☐☐ ☐ Keeping in touch with old friends
- ☐☐☐ ☐ Setting boundaries with our friends and family
- ☐☐☐ ☐ **Overall social self-care**

1 2 3 ⊕ Spiritual self care

- ☐☐☐ ☐ Spending time in nature
- ☐☐☐ ☐ Meditation or prayer
- ☐☐☐ ☐ Recognise the things that give meaning to my life
- ☐☐☐ ☐ Acting in accordance with my values
- ☐☐☐ ☐ Setting aside time for quiet thought and reflection
- ☐☐☐ ☐ Participating in causes that are important to me
- ☐☐☐ ☐ Volunteering/giving to others
- ☐☐☐ ☐ Appreciating art that is meaningful to me (music, art etc.)
- ☐☐☐ ☐ Overall spiritual self care

SELF CARE ASSESSMENT

1 2 3 ◐   **Professional self-care**

☐☐☐ ☐   Improve my professional skills

☐☐☐ ☐   Saying 'no' to excessive new responsibilities

☐☐☐ ☐   Take on projects that are interesting and/or rewarding

☐☐☐ ☐   Learn now things related to my profession

☐☐☐ ☐   Make time to talk to and build relationships with colleagues

☐☐☐ ☐   Take breaks during work

☐☐☐ ☐   Maintain balance between professional and personal life

☐☐☐ ☐   Keep a comfortable workplace that allows me to be successful

☐☐☐ ☐   Advocate for fair pay, benefits and other needs

☐☐☐ ☐   **Overall professional self care**

YOUR '1%'

Remember, that this workbook is not about a complete overhaul because as we've learned, that does not work in the long term. Just take one step, just one. Master that step, find your stride, and once that is part of everyday life take another one. Think of it as your 1%.

Newton's law of inertia states that a body in a resting state will not move but when we apply just a little bit of force, this causes movement and the form will continue to move in the required direction. If we apply this to our own lives, a simple 1% more today than yesterday puts us in motion towards a new direction.

A complete overhaul doesn't provide this, but mastering each step you take will certainly get you to your goal. It may seem to take longer but how long has it taken you to get this point where enough is enough? And so, if you only did one thing from this program. Just one step. You'll be heading in the right direction.

WHAT CAN YOU DO TODAY TO TAKE CARE OF YOUR WELLBEING THAT'S 1% MORE THAN YESTERDAY?

LET THE JOURNEY BEGIN!

In the traditional way, I place this information at your feet. If you should find something good in it, pick it up and walk with it because it now belongs to you. We do this with gifts of this nature because we understand that each person has their own free will. With that free will comes a responsibility for this gift of life that is ours. Each person must take the initiative and be an active participant to his or her well-being.

The symbolic laying at your feet shows that you have to take it upon yourself to pick up and use this information. Like any other medication, this only work if you take it.

Ralph P. Brown (Tawennihake)

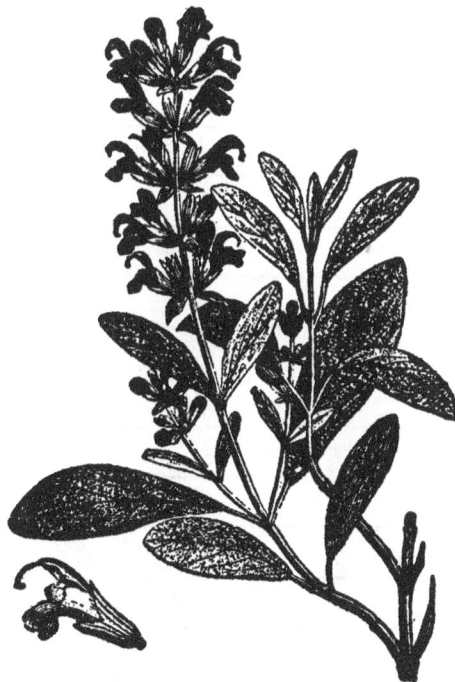

MY NOTES

MY NOTES

RECOMMENDED READING

Want to keep learning about how a non-diet approach can change your life? Here are some game-changing books to keep you learning!

Intuitive Eating-A Revolutionary Program that Works
- by Elyse Resch and Evelyn Tribole

Health at Every Size: The Surprising Truth about Your Weight:
- by Linda Bacon

Body Respect:
- by Linda bacon and Lucy Aphramore

Body Kindness: Transform Your Health from the Inside Out--And Never Say Diet Again:
- by Rebecca Scritchfield

If Not Dieting Then What?
- by Rick Kausman

The F** it Diet
- by Caroline Dooner

Just Eat It - How Intuitive Eating Can Help You Get Your Shit Together Around Food
- by Laura Thomas

Eat What You Love, Love What You Eat:
- by Dr. Michelle May

Anti Diet. :
- by Christy Harrison

Raising Body Confident Kids: A Practical Workbook for Parents
- by Emma Wright

Food is Not Medicine
- by Dr. Joshua Wolrich

The Body is Not an Apology
- Sonya Renee Taylor

EMPOWERED EATING

Awareness
JOURNAL

Goals:

From _____ to _____

date/time	what	where	Hunger level	Mindful scale	Triggers/thoughts

notes

EMPOWERED EATING

Awareness
JOURNAL

Goals:

From _____ to _____

date/time	what	where	Hunger level	Mindful scale	Triggers/thoughts

notes

EMPOWERED EATING

Awareness
JOURNAL

Goals:

From _____ to _____

date/time	what	where	Hunger level	Mindful scale	Triggers/thoughts

notes

EMPOWERED EATING

Awareness

JOURNAL

Goals:

From _____ to _____

date/time	what	where	Hunger level	Mindful scale	Triggers/thoughts

notes

EMPOWERED EATING

Awareness

JOURNAL

Goals:

From _____ to _____

date/time	what	where	Hunger level	Mindful scale	Triggers/thoughts

notes

EMPOWERED EATING

Awareness

JOURNAL

Goals:

From _____ to _____

date/time	what	where	Hunger level	Mindful scale	Triggers/thoughts

notes

EMPOWERED EATING

Awareness

JOURNAL

Goals:

From _____ to _____

date/time	what	where	Hunger level	Mindful scale	Triggers/thoughts

notes

EMPOWERED EATING

Awareness
JOURNAL

Goals:

From _____ to _____

date/time	what	where	Hunger level	Mindful scale	Triggers/thoughts

notes

Day 1

VEGGIES AND FRUIT

PROTEIN SOURCES

HEALTHY FATS

FIBRE SOURCES

CARB SOURCES

FERMENTED FOODS

ONE ACT OF SELF CARE

TODAY I AM GRATEFUL FOR

Day 2

VEGGIES AND FRUIT

PROTEIN SOURCES

HEALTHY FATS

FIBRE SOURCES

CARB SOURCES

FERMENTED FOODS

ONE ACT OF SELF CARE

TODAY I AM GRATEFUL FOR

Day 3

VEGGIES AND FRUIT	PROTEIN SOURCES

HEALTHY FATS	FIBRE SOURCES

CARB SOURCES	FERMENTED FOODS

ONE ACT OF SELF CARE

TODAY I AM GRATEFUL FOR

Day 4

VEGGIES AND FRUIT	PROTEIN SOURCES

HEALTHY FATS	FIBRE SOURCES

CARB SOURCES	FERMENTED FOODS

ONE ACT OF SELF CARE

TODAY I AM GRATEFUL FOR

Day 5

VEGGIES AND FRUIT	PROTEIN SOURCES

HEALTHY FATS	FIBRE SOURCES

CARB SOURCES	FERMENTED FOODS

ONE ACT OF SELF CARE

TODAY I AM GRATEFUL FOR

Day 6

VEGGIES AND FRUIT	PROTEIN SOURCES

HEALTHY FATS	FIBRE SOURCES

CARB SOURCES	FERMENTED FOODS

ONE ACT OF SELF CARE

TODAY I AM GRATEFUL FOR

Day 7

VEGGIES AND FRUIT	PROTEIN SOURCES

HEALTHY FATS	FIBRE SOURCES

CARB SOURCES	FERMENTED FOODS

ONE ACT OF SELF CARE

TODAY I AM GRATEFUL FOR

Day 8

VEGGIES AND FRUIT	PROTEIN SOURCES

HEALTHY FATS	FIBRE SOURCES

CARB SOURCES	FERMENTED FOODS

ONE ACT OF SELF CARE

TODAY I AM GRATEFUL FOR

Day ___

VEGGIES AND FRUIT	PROTEIN SOURCES

HEALTHY FATS	FIBRE SOURCES

CARB SOURCES	FERMENTED FOODS

ONE ACT OF SELF CARE

TODAY I AM GRATEFUL FOR

Day ___

VEGGIES AND FRUIT	PROTEIN SOURCES

HEALTHY FATS	FIBRE SOURCES

CARB SOURCES	FERMENTED FOODS

ONE ACT OF SELF CARE

TODAY I AM GRATEFUL FOR

MOVING FORWARD

As you move through the remainder of this course and finish up the program, I want you to know that I am here for you and available for ongoing support.

Whether you'd like more support working through the Empowered Eating principles through our 1:1 coaching programmes or would like to speak to a like-minded physician, dietician, psychologist, therapist or fitness professional. Just get in touch!

Thank you for your time, attention, openness and effort!

I wish you well and welcome you to contact me at any time.

Sincerely yours,
Michelle Yandle

www.michelleyandle.com
michelle@michelleyandle.com
www.facebook.com/michelle.m.yandle
www.instagram.com/michelle.m.yandle
www.linkedin.com/michelleyandlenutrition

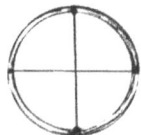

The Centre for
Empowered Eating

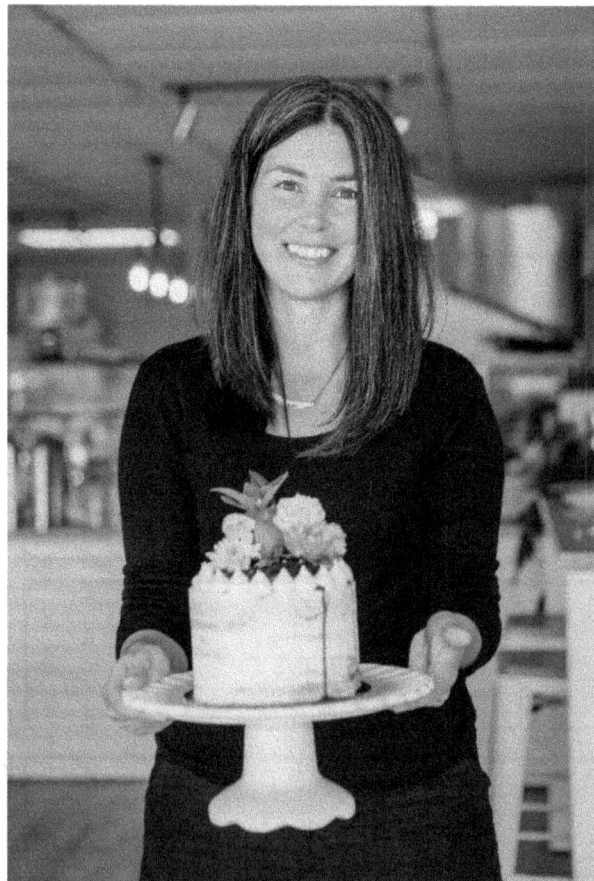

www.ingramcontent.com/pod-product-compliance
Lightning Source LLC
Chambersburg PA
CBHW080249030426

42334CB00023BA/2752